DAVID C. BARROWS

TIMETABLES

Structuring the Passage of Time
in Hospital Treatment and Other Careers

An advanced study in sociology

TIMETABLES

*Structuring the Passage of Time
in Hospital Treatment and Other Careers*

JULIUS A. ROTH

University of California, Davis

THE **BOBBS-MERRILL** COMPANY, INC.
A SUBSIDIARY OF HOWARD W. SAMS & CO., INC.
Publishers • INDIANAPOLIS • NEW YORK

ROBERT MC GINNIS
Consulting Editor
Cornell University

Contents

Preface

Just one half-year after getting my Ph.D. and a few months after starting my first full-time professional job, I was faced with a long and uncertain stretch in a tuberculosis hospital. My disease was not a complete surprise. I had been under observation for tuberculosis for many years, and my condition, although never serious up to this point, had apparently been somewhat unstable. During the course of my schooling I had already spent two long periods in hospitals for observation and rest. Now, with a more frankly active disease than I had had before, it looked as if my career were going to suffer another interruption.

However, during the latter part of my graduate career, my main focus of interest had been the sociology and social psychology of institutions and occupations. Rather than an interruption of my career, a period of hospitalization might be viewed as a research opportunity. A hospital bed would make a good observation post. I was encouraged in this endeavor by Everett C. Hughes and David Riesman, who urged me to keep a regular journal of my observations and to send copies to them to read and comment on. I kept shorthand notes from my first day in the hospital and, on the basis of these notes, wrote a report, which I sent out every week or two.

I started my observations with the more obvious and objective points—the layout of the hospital, the formal system of rules and procedures as they were given to me both in writing and in more or less formal statements, the daily round of the patients. When, after a week, I was moved to a large open room in the active treatment section, I began to set aside blocks of time for making special observations on issues that were amenable to concentrated recording. For example, I spent a number of days recording the conversations of my roommates. I spent a number of days keeping a record of the protective clothing worn by various staff members after I became aware of the differentials in the use of protective clothing. I spent some days keeping precise records on the activities of specific room-mates after I realized that the control of the patient's activity was one of the major foci for conflict between patients and staff.

As time went on and I recognized more and more of the issues important to patients and also to some extent the staff, I expanded the breadth of my observations so as to gather details on a variety of "significant issues," guided in part by my study of the sociology of institutions and the sociology of work.

I did not confide my research interests or the fact that I was recording observations to any of the patients or staff. They observed me writing frequently, but assumed that I was pursuing my academic studies. In general, my relationship with other patients and with staff members was similar to that of most patients.

I left the first hospital after three months, and a few days later I entered a second hospital closer to my home. Although I made the change from one hospital to another for personal reasons, the change also proved helpful from a research viewpoint. The two hospitals were quite similar in terms of treatment methods and medical and nursing services offered,[1] but they did differ in some of the details of their operation. Such differences were helpful to me in separating the unique aspects of a given hospital from those aspects that were more common to a tuberculosis treatment situation. My field notes, which on many issues had begun to sound rather repetitive at the end of my three-month stretch in the first hospital, now took a new lease on life as I began to describe a somewhat new situation.

Again I did not take any of my fellow patients into my confidence concerning my research interests. I did, however, tell my supervising physician after I had been there several weeks, because she was a former tuberculosis patient and had much more knowledge and con-cern about the social and psychological condition of the hospitalized patient than one usually finds in a hospital staff member. Her sup-port proved quite helpful. She called my attention to some ideas I had overlooked, especially interpretations of staff relations from the

---

[1] Details on the hospitals observed are given in the chart on pp. x-xi.

staff point of view. She always encouraged me in my research, even when she realized that some of my conclusions disagreed with her own. She also perceived that my research activity helped to make my hospital stay more tolerable for me.

My journal had again tended to become rather dull and repetitive by the time I had chest surgery four months later. Although I found the postsurgical period traumatic, from a research viewpoint it had the advantage of bringing forth a fresh area to explore. By the time this topic and the later concern with discharge from the hospital were worn thin, I was on my way out.

Even though I had succeeded in getting more information about the staff viewpoint than most patients ever get, my observations—and my subsequent organized write-ups—were still largely a patient's-eye view. I needed an opportunity to see the situation from the viewpoint of the various staff groups and to look at the whole operation in terms of a system of interaction among various groups in a hospital treatment setting. A research proposal intended to help fill these lacunae in my observations was submitted to the National Institutes of Health, and a grant[2] was subsequently made. About a year after I had been released from the hospital, I embarked on a new series of observations of tuberculosis treatment, this time as a sociological observer.

This phase of the study involved two hospitals in a medium-sized city, one with about two hundred patients treating only tuberculosis, the other a forty-bed TB unit in a large general hospital.[3] I carried on my observations in these two hospitals over a period of almost two years. During the first year, I spent a great deal of time in both hospitals, visiting them five, six, and occasionally seven days a week. During the second year, I gradually reduced the amount of observation and concentrated on areas where my information was limited.

[2] Research Grant No. E-1477 from the National Institute of Allergy and Infectious Diseases to the Committee on Human Development, University of Chicago. Grant No. RG 9813 from the National Institute of General Medical Sciences to the School of Social Work, Columbia University, later permitted me to complete work on this manuscript.

[3] Details in chart on pp. x-xi.

CHARACTERISTICS OF HOSPITALS OBSERVED

| HOSPITAL | Position of Observer | Approx. No. of Patients | ATTRIBUTES OF HOSPITAL AND STAFF | | | | ATTRIBUTES OF PATIENTS | | | | |
			Control	Location	Physicians	Nurses	Sex	Resi- dence	Race	Social Class	Age
Makawer ...	Patient	200	Govt. free care	100 mi. from large city	5 full-time, plus part-time surgeon and consultants	Registered nurses in charge of wards. Most of work done by male and female aides	Male	Most from large urban area	Approx. 50% Negro	Wide range, weighted toward lower status	Most in 20's and 30's. Some in 50's and older
Hamilton ..	Patient	300	Govt. free care	Large city, in medical center	10 to 12, mostly foreigners, plus consultants	RN in charge of wards during day. Practical nurses on most wards evening and night. Most of nursing duties by PNs and aides	Both, but 80– 85% male	Large city	Approx. 50% Negro, some Latin Amer. and Ori- entals	Heavily weighted with lower class Latin Amer. have a wider range with some in teens and 20's.	Non- Latin White males al- most all in 40's or older. Women, Negroes and

Dover ...... Social science observer	200	Local govt., means test but free for most patients	Medium sized city	2 to 4 regular staff, mostly foreigners, plus part-time surgeon and 1 or 2 consultants. Some turnover	20 RN, 10 PN, 40 male and female aides	2/3 male, 1/3 female	Medium sized city	Whites outnumber Negroes 2 or 3 to 1	Wide spread from lowest to upper middle, but weighted to lower end	Same as Hamilton
Valentine .. Social science observer	40	TB unit in large govt. general hospital	Medium sized city	1 chief and 2 residents plus consultants. New residents every three months.	6 to 7 RN. 6 to 7 aides, mostly male	Male, occasionally 1 or 2 females	Medium sized city and surrounding small town and rural area	Approx. 50% Negro	Wide range, weighted toward lower status	Most in 20's and 30's. Some in 50's and older
Sunny ...... Patient	60	Private, some patient's care provided by VA	Large city	Medical director only	Approx. 15 RN, PN, and undergrad. nurses	Both, males in slight majority most of time	Urban area	White	Private patients mostly middle class, veterans variable	Wide range, veterans almost all in 20's or 30's.

The two hospitals were close to one another and both of them were close to my home, which made movement to them and back and forth between them quite convenient. I varied the times of my observation so that I observed samples of all times of the day and night and of weekends and weekdays. At certain times my presence was quite regular; for example, I missed only one Friday morning therapy conference at the TB hospital during the course of an entire year and accompanied the director on his weekly rounds nearly as often.

In this same hospital I spent much of my time on the wards, sometimes with patients, sometimes with nursing staff. I made a particular effort to follow up any incidents that upset or threatened normal or expected procedure and tried to get the viewpoints of all concerned. I did a particularly close follow-up of a group of forty patients admitted after I first started my observations and continued my follow-up until they were discharged, except in the case of a few who were still patients when I left. For this group I kept more detailed records, including dates on which various things happened to them or on which decisions were made by them or about them, and questioned the physicians and other staff more closely and in more detail about their treatment of these patients. On a larger group of patients I kept somewhat less detailed data on such things as times of admission and discharge, numbers of passes given, and the times when certain treatment measures were instituted.

In the forty-bed unit I spent much less time with the patients and much more with the staff. Here I attended staff conferences, clinical conferences, meetings among the physicians and among the nurses, physicians' individual conferences with patients, and doctors' rounds. Frequently I merely sat at the nurses' station observing the routine and listening to the comments.

I accumulated information about several other hospitals. In three, including one private hospital, I had been a patient at an earlier time. In three others I spent from two to three weeks gathering information on selected topics. These contribute relatively little to this book, except the private hospital from which I have drawn several illustrations and which is described in the foregoing chart.

A major problem that faced me as my field work drew to a close was the task of classifying the massive field notes I had accumulated. With the help of some suggestions from Howard S. Becker, I constructed an index along the lines in which I believed I would eventually want to write up my materials, read through and indexed all my field notes, and, finally, dictated brief summaries of sections of my field notes with page numbers and index code numbers attached. After this task had been completed, I was able to collect in one relatively small pile all the summary statements concerning given topics and use these as a basis for organizing and writing a report. Whenever the summary statements did not provide the necessary detail on some point, the date and page number referred me back to the complete field notes.

I sent copies of the initial draft of this manuscript to a list of interested physicians, nursing personnel, social workers, patients, and ex-patients whom I had met during the course of my field work. Most of them returned comments, sometimes quite detailed, and these comments were useful to me in revising my manuscript. For help in carrying out my study and in making useful comments on some of my early drafts, I must particularly thank Dr. Charles E. Andrews, Associate Professor of Medicine, West Virginia University, and Dr. Marjorie M. Pyle, Chief of Medicine, Chicago State Tuberculosis Sanitarium. It should be pointed out that they did not always agree with my interpretations.

I also sent copies of successive drafts to a number of my professional colleagues. My exchanges with Erving Goffman, Fred Davis, and Everett Hughes were particularly useful in giving me ideas about different ways of looking at my materials and comparisons that I could make with other people's work. Valuable editorial suggestions were given me by Harold Wilensky, Eliot Freidson, and Elizabeth M. Eddy.

That, very briefly, is the timetable of a researcher from the more or less accidental inception of a study to the production of a published manuscript. An objective outsider with more detailed information on the history of this study might very well be able to fit it into the scheme of the career timetable that is set forth in the body of this work.

JULIUS A. ROTH

July 1963

Introduction

A patient sat outside the X-ray room of a tuberculosis hospital. "You know," he said to the man next to him, "I was supposed to get this X-ray five days ago, but somebody slipped up. You have to keep after these people or else they forget all about you. When there is a delay in your X-ray once, it's passed along to the next time, and so on. It means you get out of this goddam place that much later. *Every day an X-ray is delayed is another day out of your life.*"

The TB patient conceives of his treatment largely in terms of putting in time rather than in terms of the changes that occur in his lungs. This is analogous to the student who thinks of his education, not in terms of increasing knowledge and understanding, but in terms of the number of courses completed or the number of years of schooling he has put in. This way of thinking about one's progress is not explained by describing the patient or student as perverse or ignorant, but, rather, it is a consequence of the context in which such progress takes place. One goal of this book is to show how a person is led to define his career in terms of such conceptions of time.

A patient who enters the hospital with the idea that the treatment of TB is for a short and fairly definite period of time soon learns his mistake. Staff members emphasize the great length of time of the treatment and refuse to be pinned down to a precise estimate of just how long it will take. That this is not mere staff propaganda quickly becomes evident when the patient talks to other patients who have been there for many months—sometimes years—and are still not sure when they will be discharged. Much of the joking of his buddies is about the long and uncertain period of hospitalization: "Don't worry about who the Democrats will run for governor in 1964—you'll still be on Ward 4E then"; "The jailbirds got it better than we do—they at least know when they're getting out." The doctors tell him not to ask about his condition every few days or every week; they cannot detect any change in that short a period of time. The very fact that checkups are one, two, or even three months apart forces the patient to think in terms of a long time span.[1]

The first impression one gets of the TB patients' concern with time is that everyone is frantically trying to find out how long *he* is in for. The new patient questions the doctors, nurses, and other hospital personnel in an effort to discover how many years, months, and days it will take *him* to be cured. He asks his fellow patients how long they have been in the hospital, what their condition was and is, what treatment they have received, and how much longer they think they will have to stay. He compares his case with those of his ward mates, other patients who visit the ward, patients who have left the hospital (about whom stories are told by the remaining patients) in an effort to find which of them has a condition and treatment regimen that most closely approximates his own, and therefore, about what time in the future he can expect given phases of treatment and discharge from the hospital. Although his search becomes less frantic after he has been in the hospital for a time, he never stops watching for clues that may help him guess what stage of the treatment process he has reached and how much longer it will take.

Although there are some men without families who have "found a home" in the hospital, the great majority of patients are anxious to get out as soon as possible. To gain this end they put pressure on

[1] Convalescent polio patients and their families learn to think in long and uncertain time spans in much the same way. See Fred Davis, "Definitions of Time and Recovery in Paralytic Polio Convalescence," *American Journal of Sociology*, 61 (May, 1956), 582-87.

the doctor to allow them more activities, to get a promotion to a higher class (if the hospital has a classification system),[2] to get surgery if they need it, and finally, to be discharged from the hospital. They almost always feel that the treatment is longer than is necessary and often suspect the doctors of keeping them for an additional period to experiment on them. They count the days to their hoped-for discharge and give much attention to the actual and expected discharges of their fellow patients. And if they are sufficiently upset about the length of time the treatment is taking or any other aspect of their hospital life, they can always end the treatment on their own by leaving the hospital against medical advice ("go AMA").

If they cannot get what they want right away, the patients at least want to know when they can expect to get it. They are constantly demanding to know when they will be promoted to a higher class (that is, a class that will permit them more activity and bring them closer to discharge), when they will get a pass, when they will get surgery, when they will be allowed to go to the occupational therapy shop, when they will be allowed outside privileges, when they will be given another conference, when they can go to the dining room, when they will start their gastric cultures, when they will be discharged. As Everett C. Hughes puts it: "They are like Negroes asking when they will be given freedom and equality; their pressing is the pressing of all disadvantaged groups for a timetable."

But it is not only the underdogs who strive to develop timetables, although they are likely to be more anxious in their striving. Those who control the careers of others to some degree must decide upon appropriate times for making changes in those careers, and if they deal with many such careers, they are under pressure to regularize this process of definition. Thus, both patients and physicians tend to develop norms about how long given aspects of treatment should take—the patients to help them anticipate their future, the physicians to help them make "reasonable" decisions in a highly un-

---

2 In some hospitals, patients are classified according to condition and stage of treatment. Each class defines the patient's "privileges," restrictions of activity, and kinds of nursing service to which he is entitled.

certain situation. The norms of the patients and physicians sometimes conflict, and the two must bargain with one another to resolve
their differences (or, on occasion, to break off relations). A major
object of this book is to describe how both patients and physicians
develop timetable norms around the treatment process and how they
deal with the conflicts that arise between them.

TB patients are certainly not unique in defining their careers with
timetables and developing timetable norms.[3] Other careers provide
ready examples of the same phenomenon. To what extent can this
kind of analysis be extended? In an effort to answer this question
tentatively, I will present some specific illustrations in Chapter 4.
I will begin with illustrations most obviously related to TB treatment: patient careers in other long-term illnesses. I will then present
some less obviously related areas beginning with those having a relatively precise timetable structure—the draftee soldier, the student in
the educational system—and proceeding to those with more indeterminate and uncertain structures—child development, vertical occupational careers, assembly line workers, and some speculations about
family and "leisure time" careers. Some of these examples have built-
in timetable conflicts—parent-child, teacher-student, boss-worker—
and thus enable the bargaining over timetable structures to be further explored. These examples are intended to show some of the
variety of situations in which a timetable analysis might be useful
and to illustrate better some specific points that do not come
through clearly in tuberculosis treatment.

In the last chapter I will draw upon TB treatment and the other
examples I have presented to make some general statements about
the development and use of career timetables in defining and affecting human behavior. I will specify the conditions under which timetable norms arise and the manner in which they develop, the function of reference points, the use of reference groups in developing

[3] The way in which I use the concept "career" in this book will be dealt with
in some detail in the final chapter. The following definition will suffice at this
point. A career is a series of related and definable stages or phases of a given
sphere of activity that a person goes through on the way to a more or less
definite and recognizable end-point or goal (or series of goals).

timetables, the bargaining between clients and experts over time-table differences, the shifting of timetable norms through one's career, the sidetracking of career timetables, and the interaction of timetables in the life of an individual or family.

1

The Timetable of the TB Patient

Invariably there is some effort by the patients to define when certain things should happen to them. The patients as a group develop time norms against which each individual can measure his progress. The norms differ from hospital to hospital and are more precise in some hospitals than in others.

In the Makawer Hospital[1] the patients believe that they should get action on their case within six months after they enter Class 3 on a seven-point classification system.[2] By "action" a patient means that the medical board reviews his case and either recommends surgery, promotes him to the first exercise class, or lets him know quite definitely how long it will be before they do one of the first two things. The last alternative is rather unsatisfactory to the patient, but it is better than being ignored. If the patient is not given a conference in the first six months, he is likely to feel that he is being neglected—that the doctors "don't give a damn" about him—and his buddies will support this view. Once a patient is slated for surgery or promoted to the first exercise class, he can make a close estimate of his probable discharge date.

[1] See chart on pp. x-xi for a listing of the characteristics of each of the hospitals named. All names used, of course, are fictitious.

[2] Most patients start off in Class 3. Classes 1 and 2 contain a relatively small number of more severely ill patients.

The norms may focus primarily on the total length of hospitalization. Thus, at Hamilton Hospital the idea has developed that, unless a patient is in very serious condition at the time of admission, he should get a discharge within a year. Since patients are usually kept at least four months after surgery, such surgery, if necessary, should be performed within eight months after admission. If the patient is allowed to stay much longer than that without having surgery recommended to him, he is likely to assume that the doctors do not think he needs it. If surgery is *then* recommended, he (and his buddies) will feel that he has been treated unfairly. "If I needed surgery, why didn't they tell me six months ago? I could have been out by now. They've just been stringing me along."

The expected length of hospitalization by almost all patients diagnosed as active TB is one year at Valentine Hospital also. A patient kept a few weeks or even a month or two past his first anniversary may reluctantly grant that this is close to the average stay, but if his stay exceeds thirteen or fourteen months, he will declare that he is undoubtedly being kept longer than other patients. Valentine has a somewhat simpler classification system than Makawer, but here again Class 3 is the longest and most indefinite class, and patients expect some crucial decision on their case after about six months.

A long-term follow-up of a group of patients at Dover Sanatorium made possible a breakdown of their expectations on length of hospitalization. Patients in the hospital less than a month on whom a definite diagnosis of TB had been made, but who had never been hospitalized before, made relatively short estimates of their own length of hospitalization. Their estimates ranged from two to seven and a half months, with a median of four and a half months. They realized that many patients stayed much longer, but they overestimated the number who were discharged early and liked to think of themselves as belonging to this group. Patients hospitalized for more than three months but less than a year thought more in terms of the average stay for the entire patient population and frequently used this average as a norm against which to measure their own stay. They made estimates ranging from seven and a half to twelve months, with a median between nine and a half and ten months. Those hospitalized for more than a year, or who had previously spent a long time in the hospital and were now back again, in most cases estimated the average stay as a year or more, with a median estimate between thirteen and fourteen months.

There seems, then, to be a tendency to make the norm conform to one's experience. The patients appear to be making an effort to make their own experience look as much like that of the bulk of the patients as possible. There is, of course, a limit to this. No patient discharged after a stay of eighteen months would maintain that his stay was an average one. A point is reached, in fact, where the patients begin to boast of their long incarceration in the same way that a former prisoner of war might boast of the amount of suffering he endured at the hands of the enemy.

BENCH MARKS

Although the focus of the patients' timetable is on discharge from the hospital, an effort is made to time other events along the way. Some parts of the timetable may be defined by arbitrary hospital regulations. Thus, Hamilton does not give a pass until three months after admission and three months after surgery and then allows each patient a set number of hours each month thereafter. At Makawer, patients are held six months after promotion to the exercise classes and nine months after surgery (if there are no complications or relapses). It would seem that, in areas where the time schedule is not established administratively, far more flexibility and variability would be possible. The patients, however, find such variability disturbing and press for norms.

Thus, Sunny Sanitarium, a private hospital, does not have regulations covering passes. However, the patients observe the doctor's decisions to see how soon after admission he is willing to give a pass and how frequent and how long are the passes he subsequently gives. These observations are then translated by the patients into obligations. The patient is *entitled to* a pass two months after admission. He is *entitled to* at least one weekend each month thereafter. And if he does not get it, he feels cheated.

In hospitals with a rigid classification system the steps of promotion become important items in the timetable. At Makawer, if a patient starts out in Class 2, he *should* get a promotion within four months. If he starts out in Class 3, he *should* be promoted within a year if he does not get surgery. If he is not promoted within the expected time, he is either "real sick" or is being neglected by the staff. Here again, the details of the timetable vary from hospital to hospital, but in each case norms of some sort exist.

A classification system contains within it a series of restrictions and privileges. Where no rigid classification system exists, these privileges themselves become part of the timetable. How soon after admission (or after surgery or after some other reference point) is the patient allowed to go to the bathroom, to the dayroom, to see movies, to the occupational therapy shop? How long is it before he is allowed two hours a day "up time" (that is, the amount of time permitted out of bed)? four hours a day? six hours a day? When is he allowed to go outside for walks? When can he get a pass every month? *These privileges are desired not only in themselves, but for their symbolic value.* They are signs that the treatment is progressing, that the patient is getting closer to discharge. In fact, many privileges are taken surreptitiously by patients long before they are officially granted, but the patient still looks forward to getting them officially because they show that he is moving ahead. A patient with two hours' "up time" may actually be spending eight hours a day out of bed and at the same time be pressuring the doctor to give him four hours' "up time."

Betty MacDonald tells us how the privileges granted a patient served as bench marks of progress in the pre-chemotherapy days (before tuberculosis was treated with drugs):[3]

---

[3] This form of therapy became common only in the early 1950's. Before then therapy was less specific, less effective, and longer, and depended largely on bed rest.

The only way we could tell whether we were getting well or dying was by the privileges we were granted. If we were progressing satisfactorily at the end of one month we were given the bathroom privilege and fifteen minutes a day reading-and-writing time. At the end of two months, if we continued to progress our reading-and-writing time was increased to half an hour, we were allowed to read books and were given ten minutes a day occupational therapy time. At the end of three months we were given a chest examination, along with the other tests, and if all was still well we were given three hours' time up, one hour occupational therapy time and could go to the movies. . . .[4]

Some aspects of diagnosis and treatment may also be used as reference points in the timetable if they occur with some regularity (or the patients believe they occur with regularity). The regularly repeated conferences on each patient's case in themselves serve to break up the long stretch of time from admission to discharge. Patients use the possible conference decisions as a means of guessing when they will be discharged. Thus, Dover patients often calculate the minimum possible stay for an active case as six months. Your first checkup comes six weeks after the admission examination, the second checkup three months after that. Your X-ray could be stable (a usual criterion for discharge) at the earliest between the first and second checkups. Then you have to wait at least six weeks while your final gastric cultures are run. This adds up to six months. Recognizing that X-rays are seldom regarded as stable by the staff as early as the second checkup, patients more commonly think of the minimum as nine months unless you can talk the doctor into giving you an earlier conference or giving you a leave of absence while awaiting the results of the cultures. A patient who is past the chance of getting out in the minimum time still makes estimates on the basis of conference periods.

It was November 1956 when she came in, and at the rate she is going now she can't see any chance of getting out before 1958. Her next conference won't be until the early part of October. Even then, if her X-rays are stationary, he (the doctor) will probably want her to have

[4] Betty MacDonald, *The Plague and I* (Philadelphia: J. B. Lippincott Co., 1948), p. 142.

cultures run and keep her for at least one more conference and this would take her into 1958.[5]

The time of surgery is important in the timetable because patients always have a definite conception of how long one has to remain in the hospital after surgery. The expected time following pulmonary resection (excision of part or all of a lung) varies from four months at Hamilton to nine months at Makawer, but in each hospital, the patient kept much longer than the expected time thinks of himself as being kept overtime.

A final series of three gastric cultures is commonly used in many hospitals as an assurance that the patient is "negative" before being discharged. These cultures are incubated for six weeks (eight weeks in some hospitals) before being regarded as negative. A patient who gets his "gastrics" therefore assumes that he will get out in six weeks.[6]

Patients with the more serious disease are usually started on INH (iso-nicotinic acid hydrazide, the most commonly used medicine in the treatment of TB) and streptomycin (an injection medicine) at Dover Sanatorium. Since semi-weekly injections are a great inconvenience for an outpatient clinic to administer, patients are usually switched to INH and PAS (paraminosalicylic acid, one of the three most commonly used TB drugs—an oral medicine) some time before discharge. As a result, patients have come to regard being changed from streptomycin to PAS as a sign of approaching discharge and observe the cases of other patients whose medication has been changed in this way in an effort to find out how many more con-

---

[5] Illustrations and quotations are taken from my field notes, unless otherwise stated.

[6] Of course, if one or more cultures are positive, the patient will probably be kept for further observation and treatment. However, since the final cultures are usually not given until the patient's routine tests have been negative for some time, the cultures are negative in the great majority of cases, and patients often regard their negativity on the final series as a foregone conclusion and see the last six weeks as merely a waiting period to satisfy the hospital's discharge ritual.

ference periods are likely to pass before they are considered for discharge.

How Reliable Are the Bench Marks?

Timetable norms are not as precise at some points of the time-table as at others or in some hospitals as in others. At Valentine Hospital, for example, almost all patients will tell you that the expected or average stay is one year, that a crucial decision (surgery or no surgery, movement to the negative section, or an estimate about length of time on the positive section) can be expected at about six months, that you spend about six weeks in each of the exercise classes, that you can get a pass for part of the day about once a month after you have been in Class 3 about three months and regular passes every other weekend in the exercise classes. This relative precision of the timetable results from the emphasis placed upon the classification system by the staff, the consistency in the decisions of the physician in charge, and the physician's explicitness in telling the patients what they can expect in the future. For example, the physician usually tells new patients to plan on at least a year in the hospital—a minimum which the patients tend to translate into a maximum—and later tells them that he tries to make a decision about surgery after they have been there about six months. Such staff behavior provides the patients with clear-cut clues about when given events *should* occur in the course of their hospitalization.

In contrast, the expected time of discharge is much less precise (see page 2) at Dover Sanatorium, and intermediate steps on the timetable are also harder to pin down. This was not always the case. Patients who had been there for a number of years and those who had returned after several years related how it used to be much easier to see where you stood and how long it was likely to be to discharge. Until recently a patient had to be in the hospital three months before he could get a pass, and then he could usually have one pass a month thereafter. Patients were not given outside privileges until they were definitely negative on sputum tests and had their disease clearly under control according to X-ray. Patients were moved from one ward to another or from the north porch to the inner part of a ward and then to the south porch as they progressed from bed rest to semi-ambulant to ambulant status, and they could make an estimate about how much time they would spend in each place. The gastric specimens for cultures were "always" taken before discharge, and a patient could be quite sure of being discharged about six weeks later.[7] And finally, patients were classified on a seven-point classification scale through which they would progress from the most restrictive to the most ambulant class.

The classification system has since been simplified; and in any case the staff pays little attention to it in determining privileges, restrictions, and discharge. Passes can be had earlier and more frequently, but the patients still are not sure just how early and how frequently. Patients are often placed on a ward without reference to their condition or length of stay—some, for example, spend their entire hospital stay on the north porch, or, even from the beginning, on the south porch. Outside privileges are given to some patients early in their stay and sometimes even while they have occasional positive sputum. You "can't count on" the gastric cultures because they are sometimes taken early in the stay of a patient who is then kept many months afterward.

This change has come about largely because the director and his consultants have gained enough confidence in the new methods of chemotherapy that they are willing to be more liberal in permitting patients activities and in giving earlier discharges. The classification system and the movement of patients from one ward or one part of a ward to another is usually ignored because the doctors believe a program of graduated exercise is no longer necessary.

These changes, however, have not been made according to a systematic and explicit change in the rules and procedures, but have

---

[7] This is not to say that things had actually happened in exactly this way at an earlier time at Dover; but this was the patients' image of what had happened and thus formed the point of reference for the changes that had since taken place.

come about through the doctors' haphazard tendency to adhere less closely to previously established procedures.[8] The nurses, following the lead of the medical staff, also relax adherence to these rules, but again, because nothing is made explicit, the change is haphazard as different nurses observe and follow the changing application of procedures at different rates. As a result, the patients (and for that matter, the staff) do not realize that a change is taking place until it is already well under way. Many patients say that you are allowed one pass a month even when one of their own roommates has succeeded in getting two passes a month for several months in a row. Patients moved to the south porch still think of this as a step preceding discharge even though they have had an opportunity to observe a number of examples on their ward in which this was clearly not the case. "Old-timers" are often slow in realizing that most patients now stay less than a year instead of the one and a half to two years so common when *they* came to the hospital three, four, or five years ago.[9]

The observations at Dover were made during a period of transition—of liberalization of privileges, treatment methods, and discharge time. A new stable pattern had not yet replaced the older stable pattern. This instability was increased at Dover by the fact that all the leading members of the medical staff had many duties outside the hospital and did not get to know the patients well. As a result, they often made inconsistent decisions that confused the patients further.

8 This is the manner in which "liberalization" is taking place in almost all TB hospitals. Even in newly established hospitals the traditional rules, procedures, and classifications taken over from the pre-chemotherapy days are written up in patients' rule books and staff procedure books, and then are largely ignored.

9 Social science observers can be led astray in the same way. When I first began making observations at Dover, there was such general agreement among patients that you had to wait three months for your first pass and could get only one a month thereafter that I came to accept this as standard procedure. Some time later I realized that one of the patients was getting passes much more frequently. When I looked back through my notes and records, I found that I had already recorded several other such instances without recognizing their significance at the time.

The word "stable" is a relative one. The patients' timetable norms and the staff actions that provide the clues for these norms are never completely static. Patients are always finding differences between what they expect to happen and what actually happens, and over a period of time one can detect shifts in their norms to make these norms correspond more closely with reality (or at least with a selected portion of reality). If such changes occur slowly over a long period of time, or if changes occurring more quickly are explicit and consistent, the patients will at any given time have a set of norms that are close enough to "reality" to serve as a useful yardstick against which to measure their own progress. However, if the changes occur relatively quickly and inconsistently, if previous bench marks of progress in treatment are withdrawn without being replaced by new ones, the patients find themselves with a set of expectations that frequently leads them into making grossly in-correct predictions. At the same time they have difficulty finding clues reliable enough to develop new norms. In such a situation the patients complain that "we don't know where we stand."

As an ex-schoolteacher at Dover put it: "You never seem to get anywhere because people here don't pay too much attention to the classifications. I've been here now since November and I'm still in Group 1. My husband comes to visit me and looks at this tag and thinks I'm never going to get promoted. He wonders what's going on. Then when you *do* get promoted to Group 2, you don't know what it means, anyway. You have no idea what additional privileges you have. You have no idea what you can do that you couldn't do before or what restrictions you had to observe before that you no longer have to observe. *It's like an ungraded school room.*"

The Pursuit of New Bench Marks

In such a situation the patients do not simply throw up their hands and say that there is no way of finding out when you can ex-pect anything to happen or how long you have to stay in the hos-pital. They keep searching for clues—the poorer and fewer the clues, the more desperate the search. They grasp at anything that looks as if it might be a bench mark in the progress of time. A visit from the rehabilitation worker makes them wonder whether this may be a regular thing and whether one may now count on a certain length of time before discharge. Only the repeated failure of the rehabilitation worker to visit other patients who are later discharged causes this clue to be abandoned. The change from streptomycin to PAS is not made consistently at a given stage of treatment, but still some patients hold to this as an important clue and try to guess their remaining period of hospitalization from this reference point.

The patients at Hamilton Hospital who do not require surgery have much the same difficulty determining timetable norms as the Dover patients, especially in the latter part of their stay. Almost all have bathroom privileges from the very beginning; occupational therapy and movie privileges are usually given early in the treatment; "up time" privileges are not used; and the classification scale is ignored by the doctors and cannot be depended on. In an effort to establish a more precise timetable, the patients here too grasp at anything that looks like a move toward discharge. Thus, when many patients began to be moved to Ward 4W before they were discharged, this ward came to be regarded as an exercise or "going out" ward, and patients talked about how long it took to get to this ward and how long it took to be discharged once you got there. However, the hospital was quite new and in a constant process of reorganization. Some patients were still discharged from other wards and, at the same time, some patients who were far from discharge—for example, some being readied for surgery—were placed on the "exercise ward." Therefore, the shift to this ward could not be counted on. Likewise, there was some feeling among patients that one could expect discharge two months after a final series of three gastric tests, but it became increasingly clear that the doctors did not consider these tests as "final" as the patients at first thought.

Bench marks for a timetable can never be done away with entirely because some degree of regularity is inherent in the treatment of TB and in the operation of a hospital. It is these regularities that the patients make use of in constructing timetable norms. If the clues become poorer, the patients are more likely to be wrong in making estimates about discharge time, about what stages they have reached on the way to discharge, and about how their cases compare to those of other patients. In desperation, they are more likely to grasp at inappropriate clues. However, whether the clues are relatively clear-cut and consistent as at Makawer and Valentine, or relatively confusing and inconsistent as at Dover and, for non-surgery patients, at Hamilton, the constant effort to develop and revise a timetable never ceases.

MAKING THE ROAD SEEM LESS ENDLESS

One object of making a timetable is to split long blocks of time into smaller, more manageable units. At Makawer and Valentine the part of the classification system in which the vast majority of patients spend the largest portion of their stay in the hospital is Class 3. They move through the other classes in a more or less ritualistic manner in a length of time that is definitely, or fairly definitely, known in advance (although there are always exceptions). But in Class 3—where they get the bulk of their bed rest, intensive treatment, and surgery—they are likely to spend a long period of time without a clear notion of when it will end. At both Makawer and Valentine, much of the patients' efforts in constructing a timetable focused on breaking Class 3 into smaller units.

The Class 3 patients looked forward to being moved from the positive section to the negative section at Valentine. This shift not only allowed them greater freedom of movement, a better chance of getting a pass, and relief from having to wear a mask whenever they left their area, but it also served as the only consistent, unmistakable reference point in the long stretch of time in Class 3—a clear-cut sign of progress. For a time there was some agitation on the part of the patients to have Class 3 split into 3A and 3B, with a different set of privileges and restrictions for each. Here again the patients seemed to be prompted by the desire to have this long, unprogressive block of time broken up into smaller units that would give them a better idea about where they stood in comparison to their fellows. When the physician refused to make this change in the classification system, some patients took to referring to each other as "3 positive" and "3 negative" and thus achieved—in part—their purpose through semantic sleight-of-hand without official sanction.[10]

The Timetable as a Measuring Stick

When norms for the various privileges and diagnostic and treatment procedures have been more or less established, each patient can look forward to these intermediate steps on the way to discharge. If he fails to get a privilege, test, promotion in class, or discharge within the expected time, he is faced with the question: "Am I *that sick*, or is the doctor giving me the runaround?" In cases where the patient is quite weak or has a fever, cough, or other obvious symptoms, the decision to hold him back may seem reasonable, both to him and to other patients. However, when the patient is feeling quite well and the doctors base their decision to delay promotion or privileges on subtle details of the chest X-rays or other diagnostic procedures that are not readily understandable by patients, the patient may well consider the doctors' action unjustified. It is in such cases that conflict over the timetable is most likely to occur. Thus, the "normal" timetable can be used by the patients as a measuring stick of their own progress ("Am I doing better or worse than most?") or of the attention they are getting from the medical staff ("Are they moving me along as fast as possible or holding me back for no good reason?").

When I speak of patients constructing the norms of their timetable, I do not mean that they keep records of the times at which they and other patients get certain privileges or diagnostic or treat-

[10] The nurses too would have liked to have Class 3 split up so that they would have more sharply defined units about which to make administrative decisions—for example, who is to be allowed to do leather work, have outside privileges, attend group meetings.

ment procedures or get discharged.[11] The norms arise through the pooling of limited and unsystematic observations from which there develops a group consensus—a consensus subject to modification with time and circumstances. According to my observations, however, the norms are quite close to the averages of actual practice. If anything, the points on the timetable tend to be a trifle premature in comparison with the actual averages.[12] Thus, there is always a good proportion of the patients who are slightly behind the timetable; and few, if any, are very far ahead of it. As a result, many patients are constantly "pulling at the bit," fearing that they may fall behind in the race to get well just as fast as the next man.

Although the average time to actual discharge corresponds rather nicely with the expected time, there is a substantial proportion of patients whose careers depart markedly from the normal timetable.[13] How are the timetable norms applied to these extreme cases?

In an occupational group, for example, graduate professional engineers, there is a conception of how far a man should go in his career by a certain age. "The engineer who, at forty, can still use a slide rule or logarithm table, and make a true drawing, is a fail-

11 However, some patients *do* keep such records, especially on matters involving their own case. Renée Fox tells how chronic patients on a research ward give some definition to the uncertainty associated with their condition by charting the course of their disease as a communal venture—in this case with the blessing of the medical staff. Fox, *Experiment Perilous* (Glencoe, Ill.: The Free Press, 1959), pp. 160-65.

12 At Dover, the only hospital for which I have precise figures on this matter, 151 patients discharged with medical advice in the course of one whole year during my period of observation had spent a median period of ten and a half months in the hospital. Compare this with patient estimates of the average stay on pp. 1-2. A little less than 40 per cent of these discharges came in less than ten months, almost 20 per cent during the eleventh month (which includes the median), another 25 per cent from the twelfth through the eighteenth month.

13 At Dover, 13 per cent of the discharges with medical advice for the same group of patients discussed in Note 12 came in less than six months (though most of these were for readmission patients whose cases, the staff decided, were not as serious as they seemed when first recalled to the hospital), about 8 per cent from eighteen to twenty-four months, and another 8 per cent after more than two years of hospitalization.

ure."[14] Such a norm certainly is not intended to include the actual career experience of the great majority—many engineers do not make the grade on time. It is, rather, a very tight production schedule that goads the ambitious and keeps them up to the mark.

The TB patient whose career points greatly exceed the timetable (and despite the new therapies, some patients still spend years in the hospital) is also a failure in somewhat the same sense. His progress, too, is judged in terms of the timetable. He is spoken of as unlucky rather than unsuccessful, but the feeling that he is far behind schedule is the same. The subjective reaction to failure varies greatly among TB patients, just as among engineers some of the failures are emotionally disorganized when they do not make the grade while others accept their inferior position with relative equanimity. Some patients regard a few days' delay as a tragedy. Others do not "give a damn" about a much longer delay—"a few months more or less don't matter to me." But even the latter think and talk in terms of the timetable. When they say they are not concerned about "a few months more," they mean that staying several months longer than they are "supposed to" is not important to them, perhaps because they have no place else to go. The very use of the phrases *should have* and *supposed to*, however, shows that they too are using the timetable norms as a measuring stick, even though they are not using them as a stick to beat themselves and the doctors into action.

What about those patients who are well ahead of the normal timetable? They are the lucky ones. Other patients will envy them and perhaps wonder how they "rate" to get privileges earlier than the "rest of us." The expression of such envy often spoils the good fortune of the potentially lucky patients. The doctor will find himself challenged with statements like: "Massey got a pass after only two months here—why can't I?"; "Dayton got discharged three months after surgery—why should I have to wait four months?";

[14] Everett C. Hughes, *Men and Their Work* (Glencoe, Ill.: The Free Press, 1958), p. 137.

"Why can't I go to the OT shop—Armando is going and he started his treatment a week later than I did?" The doctor is likely to grow weary of such arguments and save himself a lot of "trouble" by not giving anybody "special privileges." If a patient who is progressing exceptionally well asks for something "extra," he will probably find the doctor replying: "If I give you a pass [or other privilege or discharge] now, half the men on the floor will be asking me why *they* can't go out after two months. I'm afraid you'll just have to wait another month."

The timetable, then, is not only used as a static measuring stick to let the patients know where they stand, but also serves to influence the decisions of the doctors. The negative pressures of envious patients and the positive pressures of patients who fail to reach the expected points of their timetable on time have the effect of moving the schedules of the patients somewhat closer to the norm or average. The tendency is for those who make rapid progress to have to wait longer for privileges and even for discharge than they would if the doctors felt able to make decisions more freely, and for those who make slower progress to get their privileges and even their discharges somewhat sooner than the doctors consider altogether wise.

WITH WHOM DO YOU COMPARE YOURSELF?

In addition to the over-all timetable norms with which a patient may compare himself to the entire group of hospital patients,[15] we also find norms for subgroups within the total patient body. It is quite evident to a patient who has been in the hospital for a time that some patients are *more* like himself than others. He divides the patient group into categories, according to his predictions about

[15] Occasionally, patients, who have picked up some information about other TB hospitals either through being patients there or by getting information from people who were patients there or from other sources, may even try to develop some rough norms for the timetables of TB patients in general, thus enabling them to compare the decisions on privileges, time of discharge, etc., of their present hospital staff with those of other hospitals.

the course of their treatment. He can then attach himself to one of these categories and thus have a more precise notion of what is likely to happen to him than he could from simply following the more general norms.

Once a patient has had major chest surgery, he will compare himself to other patients who have had major chest surgery and will try to predict the future events of his own period of hospitalization and time of discharge much more by referring to the experience of others who have had surgery than he will by referring to the experience of those who have not had surgery. Conversely, patients who have not had surgery and do not expect to get it will not take the surgery patients as models of what may be expected to happen to them.

In one hospital, where the staff lays even greater emphasis on alcoholism among the patients than do most hospitals, alcoholic patients are usually kept for a minimum period of one year. In this hospital the fact that the patient has or has not been classified as alcoholic has become one of the criteria by which the patient categorizes himself. Nonalcoholics do not pattern their time norms on information they get about the experiences of the alcoholics, and vice versa, since each group knows that the other group is dealt with differently by the staff on such matters as the granting of privileges and time of discharge.

The effect of such categorization comes out most clearly where the patient population is divided into two sharply distinct social groups. Sunny Sanitarium had both veterans whose expenses were paid by the Veterans Administration and private patients who paid their own expenses. Because of the difference in financing, the veterans were typically kept in the hospital for long periods of time comparable to periods spent in the Veterans Administration hospitals, while the private patients were usually kept for a very brief period in keeping with the drain on their pocketbooks. In this hospital the veterans *never* applied the experience of the private patients to the construction of their own timetable, since it was obvious to them that the decisions on the time of instituting various treatments, the time of allowing various activities, and the time of discharge had a completely different basis for the two groups.

The choice of which patients to compare himself with does not necessarily remain static throughout a patient's stay in the hospital. New information he obtains about his case may cause him to seek more appropriate models among his fellow patients. When the doctors start "talking surgery" to a patient, he will consider the experience of others who had surgery and that of apparently similar (to him) cases in which the patient refused surgery in order to decide which of the two fates is the better (or rather, which is the lesser evil) from his viewpoint. If he decides to accept surgery, he will then focus his attention primarily on the experience of other surgery patients in an effort to predict what will happen to him.

A shift in definition often occurs for new patients who are not sure whether they have active TB. One female patient had been assured by a private physician that he was hospitalizing her simply for a short rest and diagnostic workup and would in any case see that she got out within three months. At first, she made little effort to obtain information about treatment from patients who had been definitely diagnosed as active TB cases, since she assumed that their experience would not apply to her. It was not until she had been kept well past the three-month limit and staff members began to drop hints that her TB might be active after all that she began to compare herself with positively diagnosed patients and—using them as a model—tried to predict what her own future in the hospital was to be like.

Perhaps the new patient's underestimate of his probable stay in the hospital results in part from his grouping of patients into inappropriate categories. Most new patients do not feel very sick when they enter the hospital. They thus conceive of themselves as having a mild case of TB. They contrast themselves to patients who have a bad case of TB and assume that the latter are the ones who make up the bulk of the patients who have to stay in the hospital a relatively long period of time. Since they have a mild case themselves, they deduce that they will probably have to stay for a relatively short period of time. After they have been in the hospital for some time, they find that "mild" and "bad" are not very meaningful categories. A patient who enters the hospital with clinical symptoms and with evidence of active disease over a large part of his lungs gets out of the hospital almost as soon as a person with a much more limited area of disease (assuming that the two cases are similar in such matters as complicating disorders, effectiveness of chemotherapy, and type of previous treatment, if any). When this realization has taken effect, the patient is likely to stop trying to classify himself as a mild case or a bad case, and instead will start making use of more meaningful categories, such as those I have discussed above.

Often treatment classifications and prescriptions become powerful symbols in themselves and cause more concern among the patients than does the physical condition that underlies the staff decision to make a given classification or prescription. One seriously ill Hamilton patient had somehow managed to get a green card (the highest activity classification) during his early days at the hospital and still had it many months later when it was becoming obvious to the staff that he was not responding to chemotherapy and his condition was gradually getting worse. When the physician, at the insistence of the charge nurse, reorganized the patients' classifications, it was decided that this patient should be demoted to a lower activity class because of his poor condition. However, when the nurse came to his bed to change his card, he resisted so vehemently that the nurse and physician finally decided to forego the change in order to avoid a fight. The patient still had his extensively diseased lungs and his gradually increasing shortness of breath, but he also still had his green card and could thereby continue to place himself in the same category with those patients who were soon to be discharged as arrested cases.

At Valentine it was once the practice to change temporarily the classification of Class 3 patients to Class 2 immediately following major chest surgery, in keeping with the restrictions on activity and increase in nursing service considered appropriate for the post-surgery recovery period. Some of the patients became upset about being demoted and viewed it as an indication that their condition was getting worse. As a result, the physician in charge abandoned the practice of officially changing the patient's classification and simply made informal arrangements with the nurses to apply the appropriate restrictions and services while allowing the patient to keep his Class 3 card.

SUSPENSION OF THE TIMETABLE

The "old chronics" form a group that is often fairly easy to distinguish from other patients. They can be most clearly seen at the Makawer Hospital, although there are also "chronic wards" at Hamilton and Dover. As I mentioned previously, Makawer has a seven-point classification system through which a patient may progress from Classes 1, 2, or 3, in which he starts out, to Class 7, from which he is discharged. At the juncture of Classes 3 and 4, however, this line of forward progress has a dead-end sidetrack called Class C.

If the patient is making a poor response to chemotherapy and if his condition is such that the staff does not want to risk surgery or believes that surgery would be ineffective, the staff assumes that this patient will have to be kept in the hospital for a very long period of time before he can be considered for discharge or for possible surgery. Patients in this state are ordinarily placed in Class C and segregated on wards other than those containing the patients in numbered classes. There is not much point in imposing on such men the restrictions of Class 3 (few or no passes, not permitted to leave the ward, a great deal of bed rest, and limitation of occupational therapy, card-playing, and other activities) for several years. But when a man is promoted to Class 4, he expects to get out in six months. Placing a patient in Class C is a way of giving him most of the privileges of the Class 4 patient (and even more freedom from restrictions in some matters) without the implied promise of discharge in a specific period of time. It is the staff's way of taking the patient out of the promotion system.

The usual movement toward discharge has almost no meaning for this patient, who must look forward to an apparently endless, or at least a highly indefinite, stay in the hospital—unless he wants to leave against advice. A patient who is changed from Class C to Class 3 or Class 4 is seen more as one returned from the dead than as one who has received a promotion. In fact, a great many such patients have resigned themselves to spending many years and perhaps the rest of their lives in the hospital and plan accordingly. It is perfectly clear to all patients in the numbered classes that the experiences of the Class C patients cannot possibly be used as a model for the progress of their own treatment.

Despite the fact that Class C patients are given more freedom within the hospital, all the patients who are interested in being promoted from class to class and eventually being discharged do not envy the Class C patients their less restricted life. They see Class C as a rather horrifying tubercular Siberia—a seemingly endless waste (of time) without any signposts along the way.

2

The Timetable of the TB Physician

The physician does not have the same desperate concern about the time of treatment as the patient has. Whereas the patients think in terms of the weeks and days—and sometimes even of the hours—when something will happen to them, the physician is more likely to round off treatment events in terms of months, and, in the case of the "old chronic" patients, even of years. He will be content if he comes within a few weeks, or sometimes even a few months, of a target date in the treatment timetable. In making decisions that establish the individual patient's timetable, he is, after all, spending the patient's time and not his own.

This does not mean, however, that the physicians do not have any timetable of treatment of their own. The patients' conception of what a timetable of treatment ought to be is not, after all, taken out of thin air, but is based in part on what actually happens to them and their fellow patients. What happens to them in treatment, in turn, depends largely upon decisions of the medical staff. In an effort to carry out a rational program of treatment, the staff must give such decisions some measure of consistency.

In some cases, such consistency is established by rather rigid administrative rulings. Thus, at Makawer, the patients are ordinarily kept for one month in each of Classes 4 and 5, and two months in each of Classes 6 and 7. At Hamilton, patients are kept a minimum of four months following surgery. In other cases, the regularity is established by the frequently repeated procedures of the staff. Thus, in most hospitals, each patient is brought up for a therapy conference at regularly repeated intervals, and some decision is made about the disposition of his case, if it is only to continue doing the same thing that the staff has already been doing in the form of treatment. At Valentine, the patients' notion that they should get some crucial decision after being there about six months is not simply a fantasy that they have produced but is clearly based upon the fact that the physician in charge has given them to understand that around the six-month point he tries to make a decision about whether or not they should have surgery, or whether or not some other shift in the course of treatment should be instituted. At Makawer, the physicians have not been quite so explicit, but the patients can readily observe that in the great majority of cases a crucial decision *is* made by the staff and its consultants near the six-month point of treatment.

Such regular procedures in themselves imply a conception on the part of the staff about when certain events should occur. If, for example, each patient is reconferenced every two months rather than every month, it implies that the staff believes that there is not sufficient change in a patient in one month's time to justify the work required to carry out a series of diagnostic procedures necessary for reviewing the patient's progress and making further decisions on his treatment (although other factors may enter into such a decision, such as the limitations upon the number of diagnostic procedures that can be carried out in the given time with a given amount of equipment and personnel). The four-months-after-surgery rule at Hamilton implies that the staff believes that most patients require at least this amount of time following surgery to make an adequate recovery and to permit sufficient follow-up examinations to see whether the disease is under control in the remaining portions of the lung tissue.

Some of these time periods are based on the physician's knowledge of the disease process. Thus, the six-months' point of treatment is frequently chosen as a time for making a decision on surgery because physicians have found from experience that a patient treated with chemotherapy for the first time usually has his disease well under control by that time, but the disease organisms have not yet acquired a resistance to the drugs that are used. Therefore, they argue, this is the time when surgery may be done with the least likelihood of a spread of the diseased areas that remain in the lungs.[1]

Even in cases where the time of a given treatment event is not clearly specified by hospital policy or procedure, physicians tend to make similar decisions about the treatment of patients whose cases seem to be more or less the same to them. The times for instituting given treatment procedures, or doing surgery, or granting specific privileges, or discharging a patient are, after all, surrounded with a wide area of uncertainty. The specific time that a physician chooses to do something to or for a patient is to a large extent arbitrary. Arbitrary decisions may be more logically applied to large groups than to individual cases. The physician finds it difficult to carry out the medical ideal of an individual prescription for each case when at the same time he recognizes the fact that his timing of a given treatment event for a given patient is to a large extent a highly uncertain judgment on his part. If you are going to guess, you might as well make the process more efficient by guessing about the same way each time, especially if you are in a situation where your clients are likely to think that you do not know what you are doing if you change your guess from one time to another.[2]

---

[1] Even here, however, there is disagreement on the part of some physicians who believe that surgery in many cases might be carried out just as safely at a much earlier point in treatment and thus save the patient many months of hospitalization. It remains only for a number of physicians (and a large number of patients!) with enough nerve to try this on a large scale to see whether this idea can be substantiated.

[2] Some physician critics believe I have laid too much stress on the uncertainties of diagnosis and treatment. (Some others think this stress is justified.) Some aspects of treatment are well established, at least in a statistical sense. Thus, experience in many hospitals has shown that about 85 per cent of first treatment cases will be negative in three months. In making decisions on when a patient is "ready" for surgery, however, such statistical statements still leave a

Thus, the physicians themselves develop conceptions about the point in a patient's career at which he should have surgery, outside privileges, and his first pass, and be allowed to do OT work, get movie privileges, acquire exercise status, and be discharged. In the hospitals that operate locked wards for "recalcitrant patients," even the periods of time that a patient is locked up quickly become standardized, so that both patient and staff know in advance just how long the "sentence" is going to be for a given offense or refusal to cooperate.[3]

When the patient asks the physician when he is going to get outside privileges, be allowed to go to the occupational therapy shop, get a certain number of hours "up time"—when he is going to get any sort of privilege—the first question that comes to the mind of the physician is likely to be: "How long has he been in the hospital?" Of course, the appearance of the patient's X-rays, his bacteriological status, and other aspects of his condition will also enter into the physician's decision. However, the simple matter of how much time the patient has put in is given considerable weight, so that, if two patients have approximately the same bacteriological status and appearance of X-rays, the one who has been there the longest is the one most likely to be granted a given privilege.

The ideal of the physician is to make decisions on pass requests on the basis of the merits of the request itself and on the basis of

---

rather wide area of uncertainty in an individual case. Many decisions important to patients do not even come near this level of statistical reliability. Thus, if we ask the question whether a pass one month following surgery is more likely to be more "harmful" than waiting until three months following surgery, there is no compilation of evidence at hand to suggest an answer, and there probably never will be because it is not the kind of issue that attracts careful research.

3 In the same way, parole boards give almost all prisoners convicted of the same crimes and having the same number of convictions the same "set," that is, the certain future date on which parole will be effected. The board members have no accurate way of predicting which prisoners are most likely to "go straight," and they solve their dilemma by informally establishing standard sentences. See Donald Clemmer, *The Prison Community* (New York: Rinehart and Co., Inc., 1958 ed.), pp. 66-67.

the condition of that individual patient at that time, regardless of when that patient has had a pass before and regardless of the times at which any other patients have had pass requests granted. However, each time a patient requests a pass from a physician, the latter's first question is likely to be: "When did you have your last pass?" Clearly, such a question would be pointless unless the physician has in mind some notion of how long patients should wait between passes. In one hospital that has responsibility for holding conferences on outpatients as well as inpatients, the patient's question as to whether he can return to full-time work is always countered by the staff first of all with the question: "How long has he been out of the hospital?", rather than the question: "What is his physical condition at the present time?", which is considered only secondarily.

From the viewpoint of the patient, one of the most important decisions a physician has to make is that of the time of discharge. When asked how they determine this time, physicians usually answer in terms of the results of their diagnostic procedures. Most commonly, the sputum tests are expected to be negative for a certain period of time, and a series of gastric specimens cultured for six to eight weeks is also expected to be negative. In addition, the X-rays are expected to be stable, or "stationary," which means that X-rays that are taken more than one month apart should show that no change is taking place in the lung field of the patient—an indication that the diseased areas are quiescent or inactive.

These criteria, however, are not as simple as they sound. Bacteriological tests are only a sample, and even this sample is subject to a number of sources of potential error. Thus, the question sometimes arises whether a patient is "really" bacteriologically negative at a given time. The results from X-rays are even more uncertain. Different physicians frequently disagree upon the interpretation of the markings on the X-ray plates, and in fact, the same physician sometimes disagrees with his own interpretation given at a different time. Determining whether or not the X-rays of a given patient have or have not changed over a period of time may depend upon the observation of extremely minute and subtle and often confusing details on X-ray plates.

In any case, a tuberculosis infection does not become inactive at any particular time, but is only gradually brought under control. The physician must make a more or less arbitrary decision about when sufficient control has been achieved and the patient is ready for discharge. The very arbitrariness of this decision is probably one of the reasons that decisions on discharge in TB hospitals are usually made by medical staffs or boards acting as a group rather than by individual physicians, because in this way they can pool their guesses, spread the responsibility, and perhaps maximize justice.

The physicians deal with uncertainty in much the same way as the patients do. They develop conceptions about how long a patient in a given category should be kept in the hospital, although, as I pointed out above, the physician's timetables are not as precise in point of time as those of the patients. In therapy conferences, when the possibility of discharging a patient arises, one of the factors *always* taken into consideration is how long a patient has been under treatment. This in itself is given considerable weight entirely aside from the bacteriological and X-ray data. In cases where patients appear, according to X-ray and sputum tests, to make an exceptionally rapid recovery, one can often hear the physician say, "TB just isn't cured that fast." Such a patient is likely to be kept in the hospital somewhat longer because the physician, who has become used to thinking in terms of a longer time-span for achieving a cure or arrest, simply cannot bring himself to accept the evidence of X-rays and laboratory tests.

One patient at Dover had positive sputum and what appeared to be widespread disease according to X-ray at the time of his admission. When his case was brought up at a therapy conference four and a half months later, it was reported that his X-rays seemed to have cleared up completely and that his gastric cultures and sputum were consistently negative ever since the ones he had taken on admission. The possibility of discharging him at this time was brought up, but all the physicians quickly agreed that this patient seemed to have a case of miliary tuberculosis when he entered the hospital and "we just don't clear up a case of miliary TB that fast."

The importance of length of time as an influential factor in its own right becomes especially clear when we see how a physician's decision will change in response to a change in information about the length of a patient's treatment. For example, when a medical resident presented a patient as having been in the hospital for two years, a consultant promptly announced: "That's a long time; I think we should try to get her out of here." One of the nurses pointed out that the resident had made a slight mistake on the matter of length of hospitalization. The patient had been first admitted about two years ago, but had been discharged after about a year, had spent about half a year on the outside, and had then been readmitted. Her second admission had involved slightly less than a six months' stay in the hospital. The consultant replied: "I'd hate to let her go too soon this time." This doctor then argued in favor of holding the patient for at least another conference three months later. All this time the physician was looking at exactly the same set of X-rays and was considering the same information concerning bacteriological tests and other diagnostic procedures. The only reason for the different position he took in his second statement was knowing that the patient had been out of the hospital for a period of time and that her present period of hospitalization had been for only a relatively short time—obviously *too* short a time, in the doctor's opinion.

In the same way, physicians indicate that they have an implicit conception of minimum times of hospital treatment and minimum times to given privileges and points of treatment for patients with certain degrees of pulmonary cavitation, with given patterns of previous treatment, with given kinds of surgery, with given home conditions, and other dimensions of categorizing patients.

On the other end of the continuum of hospitalization time, we find physicians much more likely to give discharges to patients with a given X-ray and bacteriological status if they had already been hospitalized for a period much longer than the average. Thus, a patient was discharged after two years in the hospital, even though his condition was not what the physicians would have liked to achieve, because they felt that their chemotherapy was no longer helping the patient, and surgery was not feasible because of the patient's physical condition. "After all, if you can't do surgery in a case like this, what are you going to do? You can't keep him here forever, and he's not likely to change much from the way he is now. So long as he's not a public health menace, we may as well let him go out." Long-term patients are often released more on the basis of the argument that "we've kept them here long enough" than on the basis of the specifics of X-ray and bacteriological data.

Thus, we find that the physicians' conception of the proper length of time for treating tuberculosis has much the same effect as the pressure of patients to hew to their own timetable norms. That is, the tendency is to move the extremes of the period of hospitalization toward the norm or supposed average.

Just as the patients' timetable norms are not static, neither are the physicians'. Physicians' timetables do change over time, and these changes are in fact one of the main reasons for corresponding changes in the patients' timetable norms. It has been very common in recent years, for example, for physicians to reduce the expected length of hospitalization for given categories of patients as a result of their increasing confidence in the newer, more effective methods of treatment that were instituted during the 1950's.

3

Conflict and Bargaining Over the Timetable

No one can ever know for certain just when tuberculosis becomes active or when it becomes inactive. For that matter, one can never be certain that the disease *is* inactive, and a patient could logically be kept in the hospital for the rest of his life on the assumption that some slight undetectable changes might be occurring in his lungs, and that he sometimes has positive sputum tests that are not picked up in the routine laboratory tests because, by chance, the laboratory tests happen to be made on days when the patient is negative or because the laboratory tests are not sensitive enough to pick up a relatively small number of disease organisms in the patient's sputum specimens. Since, however, the bulk of the patients cannot be kept in the hospital for the remainder of their lives, a decision must be made to end hospital treatment at some point. For example, the physicians in a given hospital may agree that hospitalization should usually be ended when a majority of the physicians on the medical board decides that a patient has had a stable X-ray for six months, has had routine bacteriological tests that were negative for at least six months, and has had a final series of three gastric cultures that were negative. They certainly will not stick strictly to such a definition in all cases, but at least it will give them a reference point at which to aim.

In professional-client relationships, a decision often has to be made on the question: "When is the service completed?" The professional person usually assumes that this decision is for him to make, but sometimes he finds that the client insists on participating in this decision and that the client may disagree with the professional judgment.

In the TB hospital, the physician faces a patient who is relatively well informed about the hospital treatment of TB, a patient who frequently disagrees with the doctor's decision about when the treatment should end. The patient almost always wants to get out as soon as possible and frequently believes that the doctors are holding him longer than is necessary.

In all professional-client relationships, we find that matters which are urgent and vitally important to the client are part of the daily routine to the professional person. The client may very well become upset and feel that the professional person is not taking him seriously enough because the expert does not act with the urgency or sense of importance that the client believes his problem demands.

A portion of the life of the patient is not nearly so important to the staff members as it is to the patient. Patients sometimes become furious when administrative red tape causes a few hours' delay in their release from the hospital. At the same time, the staff members believe that the patient is acting pathologically—"He's been here a year, what difference does a few hours make?" Staff members rarely appreciate the importance of time to the patient. On the other hand, patients rarely appreciate the fact that their urgent concerns are merely a part of the day's work to the staff.

Hospital routines are organized primarily for the convenience of the staff, and the urgencies of the patients must be worked into staff-oriented schedules. For example, it is a common practice for hospital conferences to be held on Fridays, and the results of the decisions made reported to the patients not until the following Monday. This is true even in cases where decisions are made on

Friday to discharge a patient, schedule him for surgery, promote him in activity classification, or move his timetable forward in some other way. Surgery for a given patient is often put off for weeks and even months for the sake of maintaining a regular schedule for the surgeon. If an X-ray is taken with improper technique, the physicians at a conference are not likely to order another X-ray to be taken immediately, but simply put off a decision in this case to the next routinely scheduled conference. A patient's conference may be put off for a week or more if the person making out the schedules decides there are too many patients on the conference list for a given week. Routine X-rays are taken when the technician gets around to it, even though this again may mean a delay of several days or even weeks, which in turn will mean holding up the patient's forward movement in his timetable by the same amount of time. The patient who recognizes that *his* time is being lost by such delays in staff action is likely to regard this as an unjustified theft of part of his life.

To show what can be done when the hospital staff is willing to exert itself, let me cite the experience of Rita Jackson, who held a supervisory position in a hospital when she was found to have apparently active TB. Her case first came to light in a routine examination when a physician who read her X-ray thought he saw evidence of a change in one small area. In less than a week Mrs. Jackson had been given further follow-up tests, including laminagrams,[1] and a series of gastric specimens had been taken for direct examination and for cultures. These examinations would have been spread over several weeks for other patients, and in fact all of them would not have been given to another patient right at the beginning of his hospital stay.

When the physicians decided that she probably had active TB, Mrs. Jackson was promptly put to bed in a private room, and medication for TB was started immediately instead of waiting for the first therapy conference as was done with other patients. She

[1] These are also called planigrams. They consist of a series of X-rays focused at different layers of the chest so as to yield a three-dimensional picture of the lung field rather than the usual two-dimensional view.

received a pass after only five weeks in the hospital, something that other patients did not get for two or three months at the earliest. Resectional surgery was performed only seven weeks after admission, whereas most other patients who received such surgery waited at least six months. Less than three weeks after surgery, Mrs. Jackson was discharged. Most patients are expected to spend about six months in the hospital following surgery. Mrs. Jackson returned to work full time at a fairly demanding job two months after discharge, whereas most patients who leave the hospital in good condition are expected to wait three to six months after discharge before returning to work full time. The time from Mrs. Jackson's admission as a patient to her return to full-time work totaled about four and one-half months—a remarkably short period of time compared with the experience of other patients.

Mrs. Jackson, of course, had her disease discovered at an early stage and was in a condition that was amenable to rapid treatment. This is not true of most patients. However, there *were* some other patients in the hospital whose conditions were similar to hers and who did not get the same rapid treatment that she did. Ray Eaton, for example, had a very limited diseased area that was well under control when his hospital treatment was started. He spent only a little more than five months in the hospital and was discharged only seven weeks after he had his surgery. This was regarded both by him and by other patients as a remarkably short stay. However, each stage of his treatment was about twice as long as the corresponding stage experienced by Mrs. Jackson.[2]

Hospital staff members, particularly the physicians, were willing to give Mrs. Jackson special treatment and to put themselves out for her because she was "one of them." They could not give such special treatment to the entire hospital population for two reasons. First, it would mean considerably more work for the staff members. They would have to spend more time making examinations and carrying

2 Note that I selected Ray Eaton because he moved through the stages from admission to discharge with medical consent in a shorter time than any other positively diagnosed patient during my period of observation in this hospital, with the exception of Rita Jackson. It took other patients an even longer time.

Length of time following admission as patient

PROCEDURE	RITA JACKSON	RAY EATON
Chemotherapy started	Less than 1 week	1½ weeks
Laminagrams for evaluation for surgery	Less than 1 week	6 weeks
First pass	5 weeks	10 weeks
Surgery (pulmonary resection in both cases)	7 weeks	16 weeks
Discharge from hospital	10 weeks	23 weeks
Return to work full time	4½ months (2 months following discharge)	8½ months (3½ months following discharge)

out tests of various kinds as well as more time in conferences and consultations. Their work load would be more irregular because examinations, surgery cases, and decisions to be made would pile up during some periods and would be relatively fewer at others. Such "piling up" of cases is much more inconvenient and more disrupting of the staff's usual routines than a fairly regular flow of work spread out evenly over a period of time. To put themselves out for dozens or hundreds of patients would mean cutting down considerably on the staff personnel's leisure time, and perhaps even on their hours of sleep. Secondly, they cannot trust all the patients as far as they are willing to trust one of their own supervisory employees. They would not want to trust most patients with a great deal of time out on pass or with activities within the hospital or with an early discharge, because they believe that most patients would not take proper care of themselves if given such privileges.

The kind of treatment given Rita Jackson may serve as a yardstick of what may be done to get a patient through his hospitalization as quickly as possible if the hospital goes into full-speed production. Ordinarily, however, hospital staffs must practice "restriction of production" to avoid having their lives excessively disrupted by the people they are supposed to serve. Such special treatment is usually reserved for patients who are physicians, other highly placed hospital personnel, or important celebrities of some kind. The number of such persons is always small enough so that it does not seriously disrupt the usual hospital routines. However, their special treatment is seen by the ordinary patient as discriminatory favoritism.

CONFLICTING CATEGORIES

Physicians, as well as patients, think in terms of categories. Physicians often express the ideal that each case should be treated as an individual, but to carry out this ideal in practice is impossible. The physician must constantly be comparing each case to a variety of other cases. He must do so, for one thing, in order to apply his past experience to the cases that he has under his observation at a given time. Even the relatively few patients he may have under his jurisdiction at one time must be grouped together in some ways for certain purposes so as to make decision-making manageable. It is quite true, as one physician said in trying to justify the ideal of treating each case individually, that even a small number of alternatives in a list of prescriptions for medical and nursing care and privileges and restrictions can be combined in an enormous number of permutations. The fact is, however, that the physician can keep in mind only a small number of such permutations at any one time and therefore can make effective use of only a relatively small number of ways of categorizing patients in order to make his decisions on treatment methods, privileges, time of discharge, and so on.

Although both physicians and patients group patients into categories in determining when certain events should occur in the course of treatment, their criteria for such grouping often differ. Here we have a major source of conflict in the timetables of the physician and the patient. When a patient says to the doctor, "Randall got outside privileges after he was here for four months; why shouldn't I?", he is clearly lumping himself for treatment purposes in the same category as Randall. When the doctor insists that this patient must wait a longer time before getting his outside privileges, it means that he is using a different system of grouping patients that places these two patients in different categories.

One of the major differences between the grouping of patients by physicians and by patients is that of the degree of differentiation. Patients use a relatively simple set of criteria. They usually divide the entire patient group in the hospital into a few broad categories with perhaps a few tiny splinter groups and will identify themselves with one of these categories. Once the patient has identified himself with one of these large groups, he believes that anything that happens to any of the patients in that group (or patients who have been in that group in the past) can legitimately be used as a reference point for determining what should happen to *him*.

Physicians usually have a much more highly differentiated set of criteria that breaks the total patient group (both past and present) down into much smaller, frequently overlapping units. Thus, the patient who has had major chest surgery is likely to compare himself to *all* other patients who have had major chest surgery, with the possible exception of the few who have died as a result of surgery or have suffered very serious and prolonged surgical complications. The physician, on the other hand, is likely to make breakdowns in the postsurgical group on the basis of such things as whether the operated lung expanded rapidly following surgery, whether there is any significant disease on the lung opposite the one that was operated on, whether the patient's disease organisms are still susceptible to the drugs being used or whether they have become partially resistant to those drugs, whether the recovery from surgery was uneventful or whether significant complications developed during this recovery. The physician will make different decisions on such matters as imposing restrictions on activities, granting privileges, giving passes, and deciding the time of discharge on the basis of such differentiations. The patient, who lumps all postsurgical patients into a single group, tends to think they should all be treated in much the same way.

The same kinds of differences between patients and physicians occur in the case of nonsurgery patients. For example, one female patient insisted that the doctor was keeping her in the hospital much longer than was necessary, and as evidence she pointed out that she had been kept on her ward much longer without surgery than any other woman there with the exception of "those two real sick old ladies." This patient liked to identify herself with the younger, livelier women with whom she usually associated. However, her disease had shown a relatively poor response to the program of chemotherapy that the staff had used on her, and this fact was much more significant to the physician than was her age or liveliness. *He* tended to lump her in the category with the two "real sick old ladies," who also showed a relatively poor response to chemotherapy.

In categorizing patients, physicians focus to a large extent upon clinical improvement; patients focus upon the activity class in which they are placed or upon the privileges that they are granted. Physicians are frequently annoyed because patients are always thinking in terms of the class they are in or the privileges they have rather than about the improvement that has taken place in their lungs (or at least the improvement that appears to have been made according to the fallible tests used). The patients are interested in recognizable steps toward discharge such as are provided in a classification system or in an ordered series of privileges. The physician with experience in reading X-rays and in interpreting other diagnostic indices can also keep in mind a rough series of steps toward discharge and thus provide himself with another basis for categorizing patients and making decisions concerning their treatment. The patients, however, do not know enough about the finer points of interpreting the diagnostic tests to enable them to do so, and the staff does not supply them with the information needed to make such interpretations even if they did know how. They therefore stick to those clues that are more readily understandable to them, namely, the privileges and the classification system. Physicians will probably be successful in getting patients to focus on their clinical improvement only if they are able to reduce such improvement to a series of ratings or classifications similar to those now used in many hospitals for designating the patient's permitted level of activity.

Patients sometimes use what might be called a moral basis for categorizing each other. There are differences between patients in the degree to which they follow the treatment regimen that is recommended by the physicians, especially that part of it that deals with rest and the restriction of activities. Quite often, those who follow the doctor's recommendations most strictly feel that they should thereby get well more quickly and be discharged from the hospital more quickly in comparison with those who frequently disregard the physician's recommendations (for example, by spending a great deal of time out of bed and engaging in much activity). The "good" patient believes, so to speak, that he should get time off for good behavior.

The physicians sitting in conference are likely to be much more impressed by what they see in the patient's X-rays, what they learn about his bacteriological status, and how long he has been in the hospital than they are about his behavior on the ward. (The consultants and the higher-ranking doctors whose opinions carry the greatest weight in making treatment decisions are not likely to be well acquainted with the patient's ward behavior, anyway.) The "good" patient may then be disturbed when he sees that one of his fellow patients who has cavalierly disregarded the physician's recommendations about resting is promoted and discharged as soon as or perhaps even sooner than he is. Thus, again, we find a difference in the expectations of the physicians and patients because of a different basis for categorizing the patient body.[3]

---

[3] This is not to say that physicians never allow such reputational judgments to influence their treatment decisions. Patients with "good homes" to go to are likely to be given more passes and released earlier than those who are thought to be "homeless bums." Patients who are labeled "alcoholic" by the staff are almost always made to lead more restricted lives in the hospital, more likely to be recommended for surgery, and kept in the hospital longer than others. But the physicians use reputational factors, especially those based on actual ward behavior, far less as a basis for categorizing patients than the patients themselves do. Nurses and lower-echelon medical workers are much more likely to make judgments based on ward behavior.

When patient Jones argues, "Smith got such-and-such, why shouldn't I?", the physician is faced with the prospect of trying to convince Jones that he is making an incorrect comparison. In effect, the physician tries to get Jones to change his criteria for grouping patients so that his categories will be closer to those of the physician. His best chance of convincing Jones is to provide him with specific details about the case of patient Smith to show that Jones and Smith belong in different treatment categories, as well as to relate specific details about cases much more similar to Jones's to which he may more appropriately compare himself in determining how often he should have a pass (or when he should get some other privilege, or when he should be discharged, or whatever the issue may be). However, it is generally regarded as unethical to give one patient details about another patient's condition. The physician is therefore blocked by his own professional ethics from using the arguments that are most likely to get the patient to think in terms of the categories of which he, the physician, would approve.[4] He is therefore reduced to using vague generalities such as "No two cases are alike." To the patient, who has been sensitized to the possibility of being "shot a line of bull" by the doctors, such undocumented homilies are not likely to be convincing, and the conflict is not resolved.

"I CAN TAKE MY TREATMENT JUST AS WELL AT HOME"

This phrase, with minor variations, is practically a slogan of the hospitalized TB patient. A small minority of patients, like Ray Eaton (see pp. 33-34), are far ahead of their expected timetable, but they are definitely the exceptions. Most patients either believe themselves to be behind the normal timetable or are in constant fear that

---

4 I have observed cases where the physician violated this ethic in a desperate effort to convince a patient that he should accept surgery or should stay in the hospital for a longer period of time, but these cases are relatively rare, and the physician always wonders later on whether he should have taken such a step.

they will fall behind if they do not succeed in prodding the physicians to keep moving them ahead.[5]

Some patients in the early months of their stay claim that they are in no hurry to get out, that they are quite willing to do everything that the doctor tells them, to wait for his permission to achieve any new privilege, and to be patient about getting a discharge. However, most of these patients who stay anywhere near as long as the average hospital stay sooner or later begin complaining about delays in moving them along toward discharge and begin fretting about whether or not they will make the grade on time. Some of these patients who are apparently so conforming and cooperative in the early part of their stay even end by leaving the hospital against advice.

Staff members are often surprised when the apparently conforming patient "suddenly" begins to make demands to be moved along faster in the timetable. What the staff does not realize in such cases is that the patient has been making close calculations about his progress all along but did not speak up until some crucial event or series of events made it clear that he was falling (or might fall) behind schedule. For example, in the early days of his hospitalization, one seventy-three-year-old man referred to his roommates who

[5] The realization by a patient that he is far ahead of the expected timetable often has the effect of *reducing* the pressure that he places on the doctors to move him along toward discharge. Thus, when Ray Eaton made a remarkably fast recovery after surgery, his physician began to grant him privileges much more quickly than he usually did to patients following surgery. Eaton was surprised, but delighted, when his final series of gastric cultures was ordered several months before he expected it. However, getting the three specimens for these cultures was scheduled over a two-week period right through the Christmas holidays. Eaton had succeeded in getting a rather long pass for Christmas from the physician. He briefly debated the question whether he should give up the first few days of his pass so that the collection of the specimens would be completed as soon as possible, or whether he should take the full pass that he was granted and thus delay the collection of the final specimen by about ten days and thereby increase his stay in the hospital by the same amount of time. He apparently had no trouble making up his mind. "I'm gonna take my whole Christmas pass, and let the last gastric go until I come back after New Year's. What the hell, I'm getting my gastrics two months earlier than I expected, so I can afford to wait a little longer."

complained about being kept in the hospital too long as "no-good bums who think they know more than the doctors." However, after he had been in the hospital for more than six months, had been turned down on a pass request two different times, and was still in the same activity classification that he had started in, he too began to make critical remarks about the physicians and about the "unfair" way he was being treated in much the same language that the "no-good bums" used. A woman who was regarded by the staff as an exceptionally cooperative patient had accepted without argument all the decisions of the medical staff throughout almost her entire stay there. However, when one of her roommates who had entered the hospital a week before she did was discharged, she immediately assumed that she should be discharged in another week and set up a clamor to have the doctor schedule her for a conference immediately. The surprised and irritated physician, who could not understand "what had come over her," scheduled her conference as she demanded, and, at least partly as a result of her noisy agitation, the medical staff agreed to her discharge.

Much of the patients' effort to move ahead faster within their timetable and to get an earlier discharge takes the form of direct pressure on the physicians. A physician making rounds, or even sometimes on a casual visit to the ward, finds himself constantly confronted with questions from the patients about when they will be discharged, when they will get surgery, when they will be promoted to another activity class, when they can get a pass, when they will get their gastric cultures, when they will get more "up-time" or other privileges. They often suggest that they are not being moved along as fast as they should. They compare themselves to other patients, they compare the doctor to other doctors, they compare the hospital to other hospitals, all to show that if they were in somebody else's shoes or under someone else's jurisdiction, they would be farther ahead than they are now—perhaps out of the hospital entirely. Then, of course, there are always those patients who, even after many months in the hospital, continue to insist that they do not have TB and never had it and that this stretch in the hospital is a colossal blunder on the part of the physicians.[6] Some patients appear to accept the physicians' word meekly, but when one follows a few steps behind the physician as I often did, one frequently hears these "meek" patients give forth with a softly muttered curse after the physician has moved on to the next bed. Some patients argue with the physician and try to convince him that there is no use in their staying in the hospital any longer, that they should be allowed out on a pass, or that there is no good evidence that they really have TB, and so on.[7] Patients frequently threaten to "go AMA" if the physician does not give them a discharge, a pass, a privilege, or something else that they are asking for. Many patients, if they stay in the hospital for any length of time, reach the point where they begin to set deadlines—"They'd better discharge me by the end of March or I'm leaving anyway." In most cases, if they are not released by their deadline, they will not leave the hospital but instead will set another deadline and repeat the process. However, the physician can never be sure that this is what will happen, and a certain proportion of them *do* make good their threat.[8]

[6] Now and then one of these patients turns out to be right, and the medical staff finds that what it was treating as TB is actually a nontubercular abscess, histoplasmosis, lung cancer, or one of the rarer ailments that may affect the lungs. It may also turn out to be something that is no danger to the patient and requires no treatment at all. Almost all patients know of one or two cases in which such a thing has happened, and this knowledge bolsters their own belief that perhaps a similar mistake is being made in their case.

[7] Some inexperienced ward doctors find themselves bested in such arguments with clever and knowledgeable patients. They may in the future avoid such patients because, if they allow themselves to be lured into an argument, they are made to look like fools in the eyes of other patients.

[8] Patients are commonly told by the staff that if they leave against advice their condition is almost certain to deteriorate. There is no basis for this assertion, and many patients dismiss such a statement as pure staff propaganda. Long-term follow-up studies of patients who have left against advice compared with those who have been discharged with advice are sparse. The limited information they offer indicates that, in fact, the number of relapses or cases of deterioration of physical condition are a minority of those who leave against advice and indeed not markedly greater than for those discharged with advice. (See

Patients argue for means of telescoping the entire timetable. In hospitals that make something of a ritual of putting patients through a series of activity classes, the patients may argue that one or possibly two of these classes serve no useful purpose and might be eliminated, thus reducing the total period of hospitalization. A patient may argue that planigrams be taken much earlier in the patient's stay at the hospital, so that the staff can decide at an earlier point whether or not the extent of the disease calls for resectional surgery and thus do the surgery, if necessary, earlier and get the patient out of the hospital earlier. Patients constantly nag hospital personnel—physicians, X-ray technicians, laboratory technicians, nurses, social workers—to be more efficient in getting their tests and procedures carried out so that the patient's stay in the hospital is not prolonged simply by the fact that he has to wait for some employee to get around to doing something to or for him.

Patients in hospitals where the period between conferences is fairly long often argue that this period of time should be reduced, so that the staff is likely to reach a decision that the X-rays are stable at an earlier time and thus discharge the patients at an earlier time. Thus, at Dover, a number of patients argued that if the three-month conferences were reduced to six-week conferences, it would be possible to reach a stable X-ray by three months instead of four and one-half months, with the result that the minimum possible stay for a person with definitely diagnosed active TB would be shorter and, presumably, for those who stayed beyond the minimum time, the period of hospitalization would also be shorter in many

---

Gertrude Mitchell Willis, "The Tuberculous Patient at Home," *American Review of Tuberculosis,* 76 (1957), 1049-62.)

Some who "go AMA" are not seen in the hospital again either because their disease gives them no more trouble or because they end up in an institution elsewhere to get treatment or to die. Some return to the same hospital after varying periods of time. (In some areas patients are punished for leaving against advice by being excluded from all hospital and clinic treatment for a specified period of time—usually ninety days.) If a patient returns to the same hospital after more than a few days out, he is almost sure to be set back in the timetable, that is, his ward placement and classification or privileges will be those of a patient at an earlier point in the treatment cycle than he occupied at the time he left, even when there is no evidence that his condition has changed in the meantime.

cases. It is interesting, too, to find that many patients interpret the "three-month conference" as meaning a twelve-week period, whereas the manner in which the staff schedules these conferences usually makes them thirteen-week periods. As a result, many patients believe that they have been set back one week on their conference and plead with the doctor to make up for this lost time by scheduling their next conference a week earlier.

Patients who openly admit to their fellow patients that they are in no hurry to get out of the hospital and are willing to stay just as long as the doctors want them to are sarcastically chided about "having found a home" in the hospital, and it is hinted among other patients that such patients are not quite normal mentally. Such group pressure serves to bring most of the patients into line, and even those who are not particularly anxious to leave the hospital as soon as possible usually join the chorus, clamoring for more frequent conferences, earlier passes, earlier privileges, and, most of all, earlier discharge.

THE PHYSICIAN DEFENDS HIS POSITION

How does the physician deal with this pressure from the patients? First, consider two extreme or ideal-type approaches.

The "optimistic doctor" at first gives the patient the impression that he is likely to be in the hospital for a relatively short time— "you should count on staying at least three months." When this initial short period of time is over, he then extends the period for another relatively short time. He feels that he is making things easier for the patient by not confronting him with many months or a year or two in the hospital right from the beginning. In many ways, however, he is making things much harder for himself, because each time one of his short time periods comes to an end, he may have a fight on his hands to convince the patient that he really should not be discharged at this time but should stay on for another period of treatment. Also, the optimistic doctor gets the reputation among the patients that his time estimates are not to be trusted, that he makes a practice of leading the patients on and giving them false hopes and false promises.

The "pessimistic doctor" tries to protect himself and give himself more leeway on deciding on the time of discharge by giving the patients an estimate of their hospital stay that he thinks is longer than it is actually likely to be. Then, if he later finds out that his original estimate of the case was incorrect and he has to keep the patient longer than he thought, he will have allowed himself some extra time and will not need to argue the patient out of a previous commitment. By doing this, of course, he risks discouraging the patient by facing him with a prolonged hospital stay right at the very beginning. Such a physician gets a reputation among the patients for exaggerating the seriousness of the disease and the length of time required in the hospital, and the patients make a practice of discounting all his estimates.

Most physicians, however, make some compromise between these extremes and often vary their approach from one patient to another according to their own judgment of what the patient can take. These judgments, which are usually based on extremely limited information about the patient, are often wrong, and the physician has a fight on his hands, anyway, when the patient later comes to think that he has been misled by a physician who painted too rosy or too black a picture of the road to a cure and discharge from the hospital.

When a patient first comes under treatment, the physicians do not know with any precision how long it will take the patient to reach a given level of control over his disease. In order to allow themselves a freer hand in deciding what the best time is for the patient to leave the hospital, the doctors try to avoid being pinned down to any precise estimates by the patients. Pressures from the patients, however, often force them into making some kind of statement. No matter how cautious or qualified these statements are, they are seldom cautious enough. When the doctor says: "It will probably take twelve to eighteen months," the patient remembers the lower limit and forgets the upper one, and also forgets the word "probably." If he does not get discharged in twelve months, he is likely to feel that the doctor has tricked him. When the doctor tells a patient he will have to wait *about* two months for his next examination, the patient marks off exactly two months on his calendar and begins to count the days. If the next examination is a single day late, he may consider himself wronged. Again, the doctor says: "*If* your next X-ray looks good and *if* all your gastrics are negative, we *might* be able to let you out around the middle of April." The patient rushes to his room and announces to his buddies: "Hey, you guys, I'm getting out on the fifteenth of April," and if he is not discharged on or before the fifteenth of April, the doctor is "a lying son-of-a-bitch."

Any statement of the physician, no matter how tentative or how surrounded with qualifying phrases, is likely to be regarded as a promise by the patients. The more aggressive patients will do their best to try to hold the doctor to his "promise." In some hospitals there is an effort to deal with this pressure by setting up rigid minima, such as the four-month minimum hospitalization following surgery at Hamilton Hospital. This, indeed, *does* reduce the pressure for discharge during the period of four months following surgery; but, on the other hand, it greatly increases the pressure from those patients who are kept for more than four months after their surgery, because they have learned to think of the rule as meaning that they have been promised a discharge four months from the day of their operation.

When the patient inquires about possible discharge, about getting a pass, about getting some privilege, the physician may reply with the casual phrase, "Wait till your next conference." To the patient, this may be regarded as a promise that at his next conference he *will* be discharged (or will get a pass, or will get a given privilege), whereas the physician merely meant that they would take the matter up at the next conference and try to make some decision about it for the future. In one hospital the busy physician would rush through his rounds, scarcely listening to what the patients said to him, often absent-mindedly nodding in response to their statements. Patients would often interpret this nod as agreement to their request to be given a pass on a certain day, to be given outside privileges, to have their conference a month earlier, or to get a discharge at their next conference. When they later insisted angrily that the doctor abide by his "promise," he would of course equally indignantly deny that he had ever said such a thing.

In addition to discovering unintended promises in the words and gestures of the physicians, the patients also find implied promises in other actions of the staff. In some hospitals it is assumed that when a patient has had a series of three gastric specimens taken for culturing, he may expect to be discharged in six weeks, and if the discharge is not forthcoming in that time, he believes he has been "double-crossed." In one hospital an interview with the social worker about arrangements for living outside the hospital was assumed to be a sign that one was to be discharged in about a week or two, and the patient was likely to make some excited inquiries if discharge did not follow in that time.

Because of the prevalent tendency of patients to search the words, gestures, and actions of the physicians and other staff members for anything that appears like a commitment to move them along in their timetable, experienced physicians become wary of what they say to and do for the patients. They come to approach patients, especially the more aggressive and argumentative patients, much like a lawyer who is setting out to write a contract and fears that he may somewhere leave a loophole of which the opposing party will take advantage. The chief of the service in one hospital started a practice of keeping a written record of everything he said to his "more difficult patients" during informal conferences, so that if in the future they faced him with one of his "promises," he could look back in the record and see whether he had told them anything that could reasonably be construed as such a promise.

Although patients pressing for a shorter timetable are a doctor's constant headache, the patients he feels most helpless in dealing with are those rare souls who do not want to leave the hospital and actively resist being discharged. The doctor, after all, is constantly surrounded by large numbers of patients pressing to move ahead and get out of the hospital. He is used to this and is forced to regard them as more or less normal if only in the sense that they are overwhelmingly in the majority. He has worked out some way of dealing with them, even though the approach is often not very successful. The patient who does not want to leave, on the other hand, appears strange both to the other patients and to the staff, and, because he is relatively rare, the staff members are not used to having him around and have worked out no routine way of dealing with him. A hard-boiled physician may take away the patient's mattress to convince him that he is no longer welcome there if the physician is willing to risk adverse public criticism should the story get into the newspapers. More commonly, however, the physician allows the patient to hang on, passing him from one specialist to another in an effort to track down the elusive symptoms that pop up in various parts of his body. The doctor may try a few psychological tricks to get the patient to believe that he will be better off outside the hospital. Finally, if these efforts fail, he may turn the patient over to a psychiatrist.

The psychiatrist is the person who gets the patient when all other medical specialists have given up trying to find a cause for the patient's complaints. It is for this reason, perhaps, that the psychiatric literature on tuberculosis makes it appear that the patients who resist leaving the hospital make up a large proportion of the patient body. However, it is the very rarity of such patients and the consequent strangeness of their position that causes them to be referred to the psychiatrist in the first place.

MAKING A DEAL

The desire of patients to cut short their hospitalization often leads them to try to make a deal with the physician to alter their treatment timetable. Physicians regard such pressure as one of the more unpleasant parts of their working experience. They often become quite angry with patients who assail them with arguments, threats, name-calling, and (in the case of women) tears in an effort to get their conferences, privileges, passes, and discharges sooner than the physicians want to give them. The fact remains that such pressure from the patients is successful in the sense that it often does get patients results that they want sooner than they would get them by simply sitting back and waiting. Certainly, physicians vary widely in how much resistance they will put up before submitting to such pressure, but every physician does give in to pressure from patients at some time or other. The job of the patients is simply to find the physician's breaking point or weak spots.

It was very common at Dover in borderline cases where the medical staff was uncertain about whether or not they should discharge the patient to decide to hold the patient "unless he beefs." In fact, a common question at the medical conference was: "Is he anxious to go home?" If it was the impression of those present that the patient was willing to stay longer, they were more likely to hold him for a longer period of time, whereas, if he had been "putting up a fuss," they were more likely to discharge him.[9] In the case of such borderline patients, the physician was often willing to give in on his rounds to very slight pressure from a patient for a discharge even when it seemed to be the opinion of the medical staff present at the conference that the patient might be better off with another three to six months in the hospital.[10]

At Valentine Hospital, patients expected to get out in about a year and in most cases got their discharge more or less within the expected time. There were some patients, however, who the medical staff thought should spend a substantially longer period of

[9] The staff often made mistakes in its estimate of whether the patient was anxious to leave the hospital. The patient may have been desperate to leave, but was afraid to make a clear-cut demand of the staff members. Since they heard nothing from him to the contrary, they would assume that he was quite willing to stay longer.

[10] Such readiness to accede to the patient's wishes often annoyed the nurses, who believed that the doctors should be "more firm" in dealing with the patients.

time in the hospital, and such patients usually thought they were being kept too long and exerted considerable pressure to be released in not much more than a year. Patient Ernest Roberts had extensively diseased lungs when he was admitted and did not respond to chemotherapy quite as rapidly as the physicians hoped. When Roberts refused the surgery that was recommended, Dr. Elliot decided that he should stay in the hospital under therapy for a total of at least eighteen months to give him the future protection he might otherwise have gained through resectional surgery. Roberts, however, felt that he had been promised a release within a year and simply would not agree to staying a year and a half. Dr. Elliot then backed down to some extent. He first had the idea of keeping Roberts in Class 3 until he had been in the hospital about a year and then holding him six weeks in each of Classes 4 and 5. In this way, he would get in about fifteen months of treatment, in itself a compromise over his original intentions. Roberts, however, wanted to be promoted immediately and spend only a month in each of Classes 4 and 5 so that he could get out of the hospital in about a year. Elliot made no definite promises, but decided to try stalling Roberts off as much as possible on promotion out of each class. Roberts' continued demands and protests pushed Elliot into promoting him to Class 4 before his first year was up, but the doctor got Roberts to serve most of his six-week periods in Classes 4 and 5 before he discharged him. Thus, the doctor did not quite keep Roberts for the full fifteen months he had been hoping for, but the patient did not succeed in getting out in the year that he considered proper. However, the mutual compromise allowed the post-hospital follow-up examination and treatment to be continued—something that both the doctor and the patient desired.

A patient sometimes can move along faster through the hospital if he gets someone outside the hospital to apply pressure for him. Hospital physicians will frequently pay more attention to demands made by mothers, wives, sons and daughters, employers, and clergymen than they will to the patient himself. Best of all is having a private physician outside the hospital intervene on one's behalf. Such a demand from an outsider may often get a commitment from a hospital doctor for an earlier examination, pass, or discharge, while the same demand by a patient in the hospital might simply earn him a brush-off.

One weapon that patients can, and sometimes do, use to get quicker action on their case is the threat of leaving the hospital against advice if they do not get a certain privilege, or a pass, or a discharge by a certain date. The physician may, and often does, counter by telling the patient he can leave any time he wants to and good riddance. However, doctors usually have some reluctance about seeing a patient leave the hospital when they are convinced that he requires further hospital treatment, both for the sake of the patient himself and for the sake of the public, who might be exposed to a contagious disease. The doctor might, therefore, be willing to make some concessions in the treatment timetable if, by doing so, he believes he can hold onto the patient for a longer period of time.

In some hospitals patients are automatically cut off from all hospital and clinic treatment for a given period of time (usually ninety days) as a punishment for leaving the hospital against advice. In one way, this gives the physician more power over the patient in the sense that he can use the threat of cutting the patient off from all treatment if he leaves the hospital—even for a few hours—without permission or if he seriously violates the treatment routine or other hospital regulations. However, in another respect, such a rule backfires on the more conscientious physician, who is now faced with the prospect not only of having the patient leave the hospital if he does not make concessions to the patient's demands but of cutting the patient off completely from all treatment during what may be a crucial period in the arrest of his disease. Also, it is generally accepted among physicians that an interruption of several months in a course of chemotherapy greatly increases the chance of rapidly developing a strain of disease organisms that are resistant to the drugs that were being used. Thus, if and when the patient later returns to a hospital or clinic, he will be more difficult to treat effectively.

A patient might almost say: "I want to be discharged by the end of March and put on outpatient treatment. If you don't discharge me by that time, I'm going to walk out. If I walk out, I won't be eligible for any kind of treatment for ninety days. If my condition gets worse as a result of not having any treatment, it'll be all your fault." No patient ever puts the matter quite so baldly, but a doctor may well read this threat between the lines of the patient's demands. To protect the health of the patient, the public health, and his own conscience, the physician may therefore yield to the patient's pressure as much as he thinks is necessary to hold the patient in the hospital.

Even more dramatic than the threat of walking out was a "medication strike" through which one patient won his demands in less than a day. The patient thought the doctors were taking too long about bringing up his case for conference again. He raised the question with the physician several times on the physician's rounds and received no definite answer. Then one morning when the nurse was passing out the medications, he announced that he was not going to take any more of his drugs until his case had been discussed at conference. The startled nurse promptly got in touch with the physician and let him know what was going on. The physician came around later in the day to talk to the patient, who stuck firmly to his resolve not to take any more medicine until he had his conference. Only when the physician promised that his case would definitely be taken up in the next conference, which was to be held in a few days, did he start taking his pills again. The talk among the nursing personnel was that the patient must be going crazy—perhaps the INH was affecting his brain—but clearly his action got him what he wanted.

Trying to "make a deal" with the doctors is a game played by many patients who are looking for ways to speed up their timetable. Often these efforts fail. Some physicians uncompromisingly declare that they will not bargain with the patients on matters of treatment, although close observation shows that they often do. A patient who tells the doctor that he will stay in the hospital for six more months if the doctor will give him a pass every week may receive the same scornful rebuke that he would if he openly offered a judge five dollars for dismissing a traffic violation. However, despite the frequent resistance to bargaining on the part of the physicians, the fact remains that many such deals are made, and on occasion it is even the physician who suggests them. Patients *are* sometimes given regular and frequent passes to induce them to remain in the hospital. Patients who are threatening to walk out are sometimes offered a pass to think things over if they promise not to leave for good at this time. Patients are sometimes promised earlier conferences to reduce the chance of their walking out. Patients who have left against advice have been permitted to return to the hospital in a short time, despite the ninety-day exclusion rule, on the condition that they sign up for surgery. Patients have been promised discharges within a specified period of time if they agreed to take another round of gastric cultures, bronchoscopy, planigrams, and other diagnostic procedures. Patients are sometimes given an extended leave of absence to take care of what they insist is an urgent personal or family problem, if they promise to return after it is over and spend at least a certain minimum time in the hospital.

Doctors prefer to hold patients in the hospital while bacteriological specimens are being cultured because they are afraid that they might have trouble getting patients to return to the hospital if one of the tests should prove positive. However, with some pushing on his part, a patient can frequently arrange to get a temporary leave during this waiting period. Occasionally, patients at Valentine arrange to take Classes 4 and 5 at home if they convince the physician that they will follow much the same rest and activity regimen at home as they are supposed to in the hospital. A "respectable person" with a good relationship to a private physician outside the hospital may arrange to be released in that physician's care much earlier than he could get out of the hospital by the usual route. Patients are sometimes released in time for some special holidays or other occasions when their actual release date is not very far beyond that. In some hospitals, patients whose expected release date falls within a few weeks or a month after Christmas may be released just before Christmas as an appropriate gift from the staff during this season of good will. (This is somewhat similar to amnesty sometimes given to political prisoners in celebration of a national holiday.)

The main difficulty that such deals make for the physicians is that, if they become known to other patients, there will be pressure for similar deals. At Dover it is quite commonly known that some patients arrange temporary leaves while their gastric cultures are being run, and patients who are not so favored ask why they should have to spend this extra time in the hospital. Many patients at Valentine wonder if they can take Classes 4 and 5 at home. The physician finds himself in a position of having to resist the making of deals with patients or having to keep it under cover when he *does* make them, simply to protect himself from still more pressure if the rest of the patients get the idea that they have found another gimmick for getting an earlier conference, a pass, a privilege, or a somewhat earlier discharge.

BARGAINING AS A DIALECTIC PROCESS

Deals are not always made as a result of outspoken demands. Much of the bargaining—probably the greatest part of it—remains unspoken, the one party to the bargain never knowing just what prompted the action of the other (although both doctor and patient often make shrewd guesses about each other's motives). Doctor and patient anticipate each other's reactions and make allowances for these reactions, often without any overt demands having been made or any authority having been explicitly exerted. The anticipations are, of course, often mistaken, and the doctor or patient may find that his allowances did not have the effect he had hoped, or that allowances on one matter had unexpected effects on other matters. However, such unsought effects become part of the information that the doctor and patient use to decide what to do next.

I have already described such "anticipation behavior" when I discussed the way "optimistic" and "pessimistic" doctors tell patients about how long the treatment may last; the way doctors avoid telling a patient he is being kept longer because he is an alcoholic; the way some patients try to appear "good" in observing activity restrictions with the hope that this will get them promotions, privileges, and discharge sooner; the way doctors in conference determine whether or not to discharge a patient in part by how they expect him to take a decision to be held for more treatment.

A definitely diagnosed patient who has "learned the ropes" does not clamor for discharge at six months at Makawer, though he may insist that the staff decide whether or not he should have surgery by that time. He has found that discharge in six months for a case with active disease is not reasonable and there is no point in getting the staff angry at him for making unreasonable demands. The post-surgical patient at Hamilton may test the limits by trying to push the usual three-months-after-surgery pass up to two and a half months or even two months. But trying to make it one month would make him the laughingstock of both patients and staff and would have no chance of getting him a pass, so he does not try to do this unless some extraordinarily pressing circumstances in his personal life cause him to disregard his reputation in the hospital.[11] The Class 4 patient at Valentine may try to get the doctor to reduce the usual six weeks in this class to one month, but he would not try to get it reduced to two weeks because that would be going too far.

The doctor may empathize with what he believes the patient feels. "If I were in his shoes, I'd walk out and take my chances," said one physician about a pleural effusion[12] patient who had serious economic problems that would increase during long hospital confinement. But the doctor was not in the patient's shoes

[11] The staff might be willing to give such an early pass in an "emergency," but it is the staff, not the patient, which determines what an emergency is.

[12] In pleural effusion—inflammation and accumulation of fluid in the pleural cavity—active tuberculosis often cannot be demonstrated by any of the usual diagnostic tests, but it has been quite clearly established that one-fourth to one-third of all untreated cases will develop active tuberculosis in the future. Therefore, physicians often treat pleural effusion "as if" it were tuberculosis.

and, according to conservative medical principles, he kept him in the hospital on chemotherapy and modified rest. However, instead of keeping the patient the usual year, the doctor discharged him after only six and a half months in spite of the fact that the patient never applied any direct pressure for a discharge and fully expected to spend about a year in the hospital. The compromise in this case was brought about by the pressure of the doubts on the part of the physician himself about whether he was doing right by the patient.

Or the physician may judge that a patient will abuse the privileges or concessions that are made to him and must therefore be controlled more closely than most in order to benefit from his treatment. Thus, a patient who is defined as alcoholic may be refused a pass much longer than most other patients because the physician assumes that when he gets out he will get drunk, will not eat, will not rest, will expose himself to cold and rain, and so on. Refusing a pass not only prevents such behavior but may also serve to convince the patient that he is not as well as he thinks and that further restrictions on activity in the hospital and a general slowing up of his treatment timetable are therefore justified. For his part, the patient who believes he has discovered the physician's line of reasoning may try to improve his bargaining position by trying to appear responsible—hiding evidence of drinking liquor, hiding violations of activity restrictions, and repeating promises to cooperate in taking his medications, getting regular checkups, not returning to work without permission—on the assumption that a good reputation may win him earlier privileges, more passes, and earlier discharge.

Because of the judgments that the staff makes about patients' personalities and their anticipated behavior, patients may win concessions toward speeding up their timetables without ever making an overt threat. A patient's surgical date may be moved to an earlier point because the physician fears that the patient will refuse the operation if it is withheld too long. A woman's tears may cause the doctor to move up her next medical conference or her sad tales about her children waiting to see her may cause him to give her

her first pass at an earlier time. The doctor may believe that such a patient needs just as much hospital treatment as the average and may not have intended to discharge her at an earlier time. But even without overt demands from the patient, the physician may find that the logic of his own conception of the treatment timetable demands that other privileges and changes in treatment be advanced in keeping with the original concession, including, finally, discharge itself, unless there is a very clear-cut opposing consideration, such as recent positive sputum tests or obvious changes in recent X-rays. The dilemma of the staff in such a case is expressed in the rather frequent confession at the point of discharge: "I don't think he should be released just yet, but I can't think of any good reason for holding him."

With this conception of treatment, the patient who has completed all the usual stages of the treatment cycle and has met the minimum requirements for discharge (negative bacteriological specimens and stable X-rays) is entitled to a discharge in the same way that a student who has taken the requisite sequence of courses and has passed the required examinations is entitled to a diploma, even though the faculty may regard him as an unimaginative bore.

The anticipation of and allowances for the reactions of the other party on both sides of a continuing bargaining system form a dialectic of constant mutual influences operating over a period of time. Some of these influences are the outspoken demands of doctors and patients on one another; some are demands and expectations talked over only within each colleague group; some operate only within the minds of the individuals and are never openly expressed. Such a dialectic cannot be meaningfully analyzed as an event or a single interaction, but only as a continuing process with an arbitrary beginning and end. The following illustration is an attempt to show how such bargaining—partly overt, partly hidden from view—operates.

Patients constantly press for advancing the timetable; physicians try to resist such pressures. But on one occasion a patient offers a particularly compelling argument about why he should have his first pass a month earlier than usual and it is granted. Now it becomes more difficult for the doctor to refuse similar requests from other patients because he is faced with the question of whether it is fair to grant the earlier privilege to one and not to others.[13] He therefore finds himself granting earlier passes to others with less compelling arguments. The more conforming patient, who would not have thought of pressing for an earlier pass before, now cannot see why he should not get what others get. Patients are no longer asking to be granted an exception, but simply to be given what everybody else is getting.

At this point the earlier passes may become stabilized at a new point in the timetable. They may even have the effect of moving forward some other privileges since the patients, and even the physician in his own mind, can argue: "If passes can be taken safely a month earlier, why can't . . . ?" The doctor may feel retrospectively that he has been tricked, but he may not consider the issue important enough to fight about and lets the matter stand. On the other hand, he may decide that the changed state of affairs is not in keeping with a proper treatment regimen, or that the patients will take advantage of his leniency in this case to make inroads on the restrictions in other areas, or that the shift in passes to an earlier point on the timetable damages the logic of the graduated activity program and thus threatens to destroy the program as a whole. In such a case he may firmly refuse to grant any more earlier passes. The patients call such action "a crackdown." There will be a period of ill-feeling while the patients accuse the doctor of reneging on his bargain and the doctor accuses the patients of having tried to put something over on him. For a time the patients will let up on their demands and their pressure against the limits in all directions, while the doctor will keep a sharp eye open to see that

[13] One way this dilemma is sometimes handled is to define the concession as extraordinary in some way and therefore not really a modification of the usual timetable. Thus, the earlier pass may be defined by the staff as an emergency pass and therefore not really the patient's first pass in the ordinary sense. However, other patients often refuse to accept such definitions and to insist that they are entitled to the same concessions.

he is not "tricked" again. However, in hospitals, as in other areas of conflict, such campaigns blow over. The patients dissect the doctor's words and actions, as well as picking up any information they can from the ward personnel and others, to find out when the doctor has "cooled off." Finally, a few of the more venturesome patients will tentatively renew their demands. The first efforts may be sharply rejected, proving that the patients' timing was wrong. But the time will come when the traumatic effects of the previous incident will wear off, and the doctor will once again grapple with himself about just what the fair and humane way is to deal with the needs of the patients. Again he will begin to make concessions to the pressures and anticipated pressures of the patients and the cycle is repeated—although things are never *quite* the same after any cycle as they were before.

Recapitulation　　1

Objectively, the period of time that a TB patient will spend in the hospital may vary rather widely and cannot be accurately predicted in any given case until perhaps in the latter part of the treatment process. Recognizing this, physicians attempt to avoid any commitments on the length of time of a particular treatment or any stage of treatment. They are not successful in this effort, both because patients often press them into making tentative predictions and because patients obtain clues about the treatment timetable from other sources, including their own observations of the regularities inherent in the treatment program.

The clues that the patients accumulate become a group product as a result of the constant discussion among patients about the timing of events in their treatment and hospital life. Such an interchange of experience and observation produces norms about when given events in one's treatment "should" occur. Therapy conferences, changes in activity classifications, the granting of privileges, the removal of restrictions, diagnostic procedures, surgery, changes in treatment may all serve as bench marks in a timetable that lets a patient know how far he is on the road to discharge. Such norms serve as a yardstick of progress—each patient may compare his progress with that of the norms to see whether he is ahead of or behind schedule.

In hospitals where the treatment program has been relatively stable for some time or where changes in the program are made explicit to the patients, the timetable norms of the patients are relatively precise and close to "reality." Where the program is undergoing fairly rapid change that is inconsistent or is not made explicit to patients, the norms will always be somewhat out of date and the patients will be desperately seeking clues to establish a more reliable timetable.

Physicians, too, develop treatment timetable norms as a way of dealing both with the uncertainties of diagnosis and prognosis and with the pressures from the patients to be discharged from the hospital as soon as possible. Doctors have a conception of approximately how long a patient with given disease characteristics (and sometimes certain social and behavioral characteristics) should take to get his disease under sufficient control to warrant discharge (or surgery or privileges or change in treatment program).

In trying to anticipate their future timetable, patients compare themselves to others whose cases appear most like their own. Physicians, too, categorize patients in order to achieve a regularity in their treatment decisions from case to case. Conflict over the time-table often arises between physicians and patients because they use different sets of categories—those of the physicians being more highly differentiated than those of the patients. Thus, the patient may expect to be treated like one group of patients while the physician considers it more appropriate to treat him like a different group.

Patients as a group, moreover, maintain a constant pressure to be moved along faster on the timetable, the pressure increasing sharply as patients perceive themselves falling behind schedule. The physicians attempt to resist these pressures so that they may control the treatment timetable in the manner they consider appropriate. The result of these opposing pressures is a continual process of bargaining between patients and physicians over the question of when given points on the timetable will be reached. Such bargaining includes the application of pressures for decision or action, threats, deals, manipulation, and compromise as each party strives to reach his goals, but recognizes the limitations imposed by the counter-stance and the bargaining power of the other party. Most of all, such bargaining consists of a dialectic of anticipation of reactions of the other party—the patient is not free *in his own mind* to make unreasonable demands and the doctor is likewise not free to ignore the pressures from the patients. The actual timetable of treatment is a resultant of the interaction of such explicit and implicit forces.

4

Some Other Career Timetables

The way in which the passage of time is defined and structured by TB patients and physicians is not unique to the TB treatment situation. Such a concept of time is part of our usual mode of thought. We apply it to many aspects of our daily lives and to our careers and those of other people.

In this chapter I will present a number of illustrations to show that the concepts of time and the interaction associated with them that are found in the tuberculosis treatment setting are employed in all their detail in other career settings. Some of these examples are quite clear-cut and obvious. A few are rather tenuous and speculative—an effort on my part to see how far the concepts might be stretched, and, hopefully, to stimulate others to carry the ideas further and to modify them in their own studies. In the final chapter I will review in a general way the various issues that may have to be considered in the study of career timetables.

POLIO CONVALESCENCE

Let us look first at an illustration that is a striking parallel to the TB treatment situation: paralytic polio convalescence as it is described in a study by Fred Davis.[1] The professional-client relation-

---

[1] *Passage Through Crisis: Polio Victims and Their Families* (Indianapolis, Indiana: The Bobbs-Merrill Company, Inc., 1963).

ships in this case are more complex because the parents of the child patients, as well as the patients themselves, are the clients of the hospital staff, and the physiotherapists, as well as the physicians, have a major role in controlling the treatment regimen that to a great extent provides the reference points for the treatment timetable.

When the acute stage of a polio attack has passed, both the child patient and his parents are very uncertain about how much recovery to expect, how much time will have to be spent in the convalescent hospital, and how long the total, or maximum, recovery will take. The patient soon gets a better idea of what will happen to him in the same way that the TB patient does. He learns from observing what happens to other patients and by talking to treatment personnel, and much more by talking to his fellow patients, that treatment events and the privileges that go with them come in a more or less definite sequence, each one a step forward toward discharge from the hospital and perhaps recovery of muscle function. He moves from stretcher-bed manipulations to hydrotherapy baths to leg exercises to standing-while-held to walking between arm rails to walking with braces or crutches. At a certain time he is allowed to sit up in bed and at another phase of the treatment is given a wheelchair.

Not only do the polio patients learn the sequence and thus know at any given time about how far along they are, but they learn to expect the various events to come at certain times in relation to one another. The periodic "muscle checks" (which seem to serve much the same purpose as the periodic X-rays and sputum tests do for TB patients) occur every four to six weeks, and the decision on making use of braces or crutches usually comes after the second muscle check. As with TB patients, the privileges and restrictions that structure the timetable do not necessarily describe the actual activity of the polio patients—they often "sneak a walk" before they are allowed to—but serve more as symbols of the forward progress they are making. During this period there is no evidence of recovery that is readily observable by the patients, and if it were not for the labeling and defining of the phases of physiotherapy and the kinds of recovery of muscle function (often obscure to the un-initiated) that occur, the patients would have no way of knowing how far (or even whether) they were progressing.

Like the TB patients at Dover, the polio patients and their parents first underestimate the length of the treatment regimen and only gradually learn to think in terms of longer time perspectives. The parents, however, never develop as precise and detailed a timetable, at least of the hospital part of the treatment, as do the polio patients because their sources of information are much more limited—staff personnel who "don't want to stick their neck out" and therefore give very little useful information,[2] other parents who know no more than they do, outside doctors who do not want to interfere with the hospital handling of the case, and a few second- and third-hand stories about others who had polio. They do not utilize their best potential source of information—their stricken child—because they do not want to use the few brief visiting periods upsetting him with talk about his disease and treatment and perhaps would consider a child's statements unreliable if he volunteered the information. During the hospital period, the parents remain in the stage of desperately hunting clues for constructing a more precise and reliable timetable, usually without getting far in this direction.

The patients themselves quickly learn to recognize different categories among their fellow patients—to distinguish the bone disease cases from the polios, the new polios (with recent acute illness) from old polios (return to the hospital for corrective surgery or other special treatment)—and realize that the times and the sequence of events that apply to one group do not apply to the others. Again, the staff probably has a more differentiated way of categorizing the patients, perhaps on the basis of the muscle function tests or the kind of corrective devices needed, though Davis does not give evidence on this point.

2 Apparently, in the hospital observed by Davis there were no doctors comparable to my "pessimistic" doctors.

Although staff members present parents with the usual medical dictum that each case is different, it is quite clear that they too operate on an expected timetable. At a certain time an estimate of residual damage can be made and the initial use of braces and crutches decided upon; physiotherapy is continued for a certain length of time and then decreased on a more or less regular schedule; corrective surgery is considered at approximately a certain length of time after treatment is instituted; and so on. Some of these time points are in large part the product of clinical experience with the time usually needed for certain changes to occur following polio. Quite often they are a way of maintaining a convenient routine for physicians and physiotherapists, of exercising a measure of psychological control over the patients—for example, avoiding the envy that might develop if some patients progressed much faster than others—and of structuring the medical personnel's own uncertainty about when and for how long given treatment procedures—for example, physiotherapy—can be effectively instituted.

There is also a post-hospital timetable in which the physicians estimate the maximum length of time in which any further recovery in muscle function may occur. Parents use this timetable as a yardstick to measure the recovery rate of their child in an effort to determine whether, at the rate he is going, he will be back to normal before the time is up. If the child returns to an essentially normal state well before the end of this time limit (which the physicians do not regard as a precise limit, but as a roughly estimated reasonable time), he is thought of by his parents (and presumably others familiar with the case) as reaching the goal in "under par" time.

Where the child makes no significant progress toward normality for a long period following discharge from the hospital, he is seen by his parents as being behind schedule, since, if he keeps going at that rate, he will still be noticeably handicapped when the time is up. Such parents may interpret the physician's statements in such a way as to allow them more time for recovery to take place much as tuberculosis patients often interpret the doctor's statements in such a way that they see themselves being released from the hospital earlier than the doctor intended.

The attending physician's advice to discard crutches or braces, to change to a shorter brace, to try out another, more demanding activity, and other progressive changes in the treatment regimen may serve as bench marks on the road to maximum recovery. Once out of the hospital, however, the opportunity for timetable norms to develop may be limited by the fact that members of the group concerned (patients and their parents) are no longer in contact with one another and therefore cannot exchange their experiences, hopes, and expectations. In places where there are post-polio clubs, such group norms following hospitalization would almost certainly develop.

THE PSYCHIATRIC PATIENT

The passage of patients through a mental hospital is a rich source for the study of career timetables. No study to my knowledge has dealt specifically with this aspect of mental hospital functioning, but some descriptions carry hints about what might be looked for if we made such a study.[3]

Mental patients, like TB patients, often start their career thinking their incarceration will be short and have a definite end-point. They are soon "put wise" by their fellow inmates and their own observations. If they want to anticipate their future, they must "dope out" their timetable from available clues.

The research reports cited give some idea what these clues might be. In the large hospitals where the many wards are used for dif-

---

[3] I draw here mainly upon Erving Goffman, *Asylums* (Garden City, N. Y.: Anchor Books, Doubleday and Co., Inc., 1961), especially the papers "The Underlife of a Public Institution" and "The Medical Model and Mental Hospitalization"; Ivan Belknap, *Human Problems of a State Mental Hospital* (New York: McGraw-Hill Book Co., Inc., 1956); Alfred H. Stanton and Morris S. Schwartz, *The Mental Hospital* (New York: Basic Books, Inc., 1954).

ferent purposes, mental patients can make use of their transfers from ward to ward to trace their progress through the treatment program and make estimates about their prognosis. Thus, a patient will start on the admission ward. The place to which he is transferred may suggest (once he knows how the system works) about how far from the discharge point he is starting out. A move from a closed ward to an open ward is a progressive step, and even on the locked ward a decreasing degree of supervision may indicate forward movement. A move to a convalescent ward tells the patient that he can expect to be discharged before long, and in a given institution even the amount of time to discharge (or furlough) may be calculable with a fair degree of precision. Even a series of shock treatments may mark a given stage of progress.

Some of the privileges become part of the timetable. A mental patient moves progressively from being confined to the ward to receiving movie and concert privileges, the right to stay outside the building, five o'clock parole, nine o'clock parole, and finally town parole. In some hospitals, being given a work assignment with little or no supervision or receiving permission to attend patient socials are also bench marks of progress. We can expect that patients who are aware of what is happening to them and to their fellows will develop some norms about how long it should take to move from one of these points to another.

There seems to be much more back-and-forth movement on the timetable of mental patients than on that of TB patients. The great majority of TB patients who do not "go AMA" move steadily forward from admission to discharge, although their rates of forward movement vary. Relatively few TB patients are set back as a result of a relapse during any one period of hospitalization. In mental hospitals such setbacks appear to be a common event in the experience of the inmate population. Patients accumulate advanced privileges and even reach the convalescent ward and then "mess up" and go back to a closed ward and start over at an earlier point of the timetable. Whether the norms for the second time around (or the third, etc.) are the same as those of the first would be an interesting question in itself.[4]

Undoubtedly mental hospital inmates have some ways of differentiating their fellows into groups with different chances and rates of progress (for example, organic and nonorganic cases) and decide which of the groups they most resemble. It also seems likely that the patients' classifications differ in important ways from those of the staff and that the inmates will therefore consider unfair some staff decisions about their forward movement or the lack of it.

The back wards of the mental hospitals seem to be the equivalent of the Class C category at Makawer—a way of shunting "hopeless" patients out of the promotion system. An important difference is that, while in TB treatment only a small minority of patients end up on the "chronic sidetrack," in mental hospitals a large proportion do—until recent years a majority. Thus, a patient who has hopes of returning to the outside world must worry much more about being shipped to a chronic service (or "continued-treatment unit" as it is often euphemistically called) than about going to the disturbed unit—the latter often being only a temporary stay while he cools off.

In the mental hospital Goffman observed, a typical sequence for patients who were discharged took about nine months. With some variations in the sequence, it might take up to two years to discharge. A patient who did not make the grade in about two years would be transferred to another part of the hospital, and his chances of release were greatly reduced. He was shifted to the "chronic sidetrack," or, as Goffman calls it, the "failure timetable." The same set of privileges was used for the patients on the discharge timetable and those on the failure timetable, but the

---

[4] When a patient is demoted through ward reassignment, he feels that he should have to pay a certain time on the "bad" ward as punishment for his transgression. He can pay back this time faster by doing ward work and attending group therapy. (Erving Goffman, personal communication.)

In some respects, the demoted patient is in a position similar to that of the readmitted patient with regard to the treatment timetable. Goffman's impression is that readmitted patients are usually left on the "bad" wards for a shorter period than are first admissions.

privileges had a different meaning for the two groups. For patients on the acute service, the privileges represent markers on the way to discharge. For those on a chronic service, privileges are amenities lost by "messing up" and regained after an appropriate period of suffering without them, but not leading anywhere except to a repetition of the cycle. Work assignments also have different meanings for the two groups—for the chronic patient, a form of custodial treatment and a way of getting the ward work done (earning his keep); for the acute patient, a test of his readiness to move ahead in the discharge timetable.

The timetables developed by the staff would also be a crucial part of such a study. Sommer and Osmond point out that two years seems to be a magic number.[5] The assumption has often been made that patients must get out within two years or they are likely to be stuck for life.[6] To what extent is this conception a self-fulfilling prophecy—that is, do patients who stay past a certain time tend to be shunted into a chronic unit and forgotten?

In controlling the patients' timetables, nursing personnel play only a minor role in the TB hospital—a nurse may, for example, give the physician information about a patient's drinking that causes the physician to define the patient as an alcoholic and thus hold him in the hospital longer—and for that reason I have largely ignored them in the earlier description of the TB treatment timetable. In mental hospitals, attendants play a much more important role, which would have to be carefully investigated in a study of patient-staff bargaining over the timetable. For example, attendants initiate many of the demotions and loss of privileges, even though a physician must sign the order.

At first sight, the mental patient appears to be in a poor bargaining position compared to the TB patient. In most cases, he can-

[5] Robert Sommer and Humphry Osmond, "Symptoms of Institutional Care," *Social Problems*, 8 (Winter, 1961), 261.

[6] With the emphasis on faster turnover in recent years, the magic number may be dropping to one year in some institutions.

not threaten to "go AMA," which is one of the TB patient's most potent weapons. The mental hospital staff may protect its position by interpreting the patient's demands and arguments as symptoms of his illness. Outsiders who try to intervene on the patient's behalf are often convinced that the patient's tale cannot be taken seriously because he is crazy. However, the patient is by no means helpless in this situation.

Goffman's "Underlife"[7] is in large part a chronicle of the ways in which patients can get around institutional controls; and some of these ways affect the patients' timetables. Certainly, acting a part plays a much more crucial role in the mental hospital than in the TB hospital. After all, the inmate has been defined as mentally ill because of his behavior and can get himself defined as improved or cured by the same route. A patient with any contact with the world around him is sure to pick up some clues about how the staff defines sickness and normality, although patients no doubt vary greatly in their perceptiveness. If a patient is sufficiently anxious for promotion and discharge, he can make an effort to "act right" to bolster his reputation as an improving patient. Conversely, if he does not want to leave, he can stretch out his timetable by "messing up."

The fact that a patient's behavior is simultaneously interpreted as evidence of mental illness and as actions to be dealt with by another party to a bargaining system may often face the patient with delicate and difficult decisions. Thus, a patient may make aggressive demands to be discharged as a way of bringing himself to the notice of physicians who have forgotten about him, but if he is *too aggressive* the physicians may simply be convinced that his behavior shows that he is not ready for discharge. Add to this balancing act the fact that psychiatric classifications and interpretations are nebulous even to the specialist, that several schools of thought are likely to be represented on any large staff, that the behavior which pleases attendants is often quite different from that which pleases physicians, and we can see that the patient will have many difficult decisions

[7] See p. 67, note 3.

to make both about what to anticipate in his future and about how he might influence that future through his own behavior. These very uncertainties and the need to deal with them, though hard on the patient, make this an especially fruitful setting for social-psychological investigation.

THE STANDARDIZED TIMETABLE

Developing a career timetable with group norms is not limited to the area of medical treatment but is much more widely applicable as a device to structure career-oriented behavior. First, let us look at two cases with a highly standardized timetable.

The Draftee Army

Eugene Uyeki provides an excellent description of the career of the draftee soldier whose timetable has a precisely determined beginning and end-point.[8] In this career it remains for the participants only to fill in the intervening time with a meaningful structure that will break the two-year stretch into smaller units denoting progress toward their goal.

Unless the draftee is eliminated by such things as disability or conviction of a crime, he goes on counting the time—first in months, then weeks, and finally days—to the end of his term of duty. An important aspect of a soldier's position with his fellows is the amount of time he has left, and the soldiers are constantly questioning one another on this subject. In addition to obvious time units, the soldier may measure his progress by counting regularly scheduled events: inspections, full-fields, KP's, field problems. "The importance of these activities to the draftee is in categorizing the two years into a limited and definable series of events with a predetermined conclusion—the return to civilian life."

8 Eugene S. Uyeki, "Draftee Behavior in the Cold-War Army," *Social Problems*, 8 (Fall, 1960), 151-58. See especially p. 155.

The Educational System

One of our most highly organized and standardized timetables is that provided by our educational system. The school year begins and ends about the same time in all schools. Children start in kindergarten and step forward one grade each year until they graduate from high school. The "drop-out" receives much the same scorn from those in authority as does the AMA patient in a TB hospital, although teachers, like hospital personnel, are often glad to get rid of "troublemakers" before their expected period of schooling (treatment) is ended. Any pupil can promptly be placed in the rigid timetable by being designated by such terms as "seventh-grader" or "high-school sophomore." It is a system in which the pupils, their parents, the teachers, and anyone else concerned agrees on the reference points as well as the end-point in the timetable.

The deviants are described in terms of the normal timetable. An outstanding pupil "skips a grade" and is "a year ahead." An unproductive pupil is "kept back" and falls "a year behind." When the conflict over racial integration closes the schools in a community, both the segregationists and integrationists worry about the pupils who have "lost a year." Foreign educational systems become meaningful only in terms of our own timetable. The German *Gymnasium* is described by American writers as the equivalent of high school and the *Hochschule* as the equivalent of technical college, although neither of these comparisons is quite true. And the saddest of all fates, placement in an ungraded class (and thus removal from the normal timetable entirely), is reserved for those who are considered hopelessly retarded.

We think of four years as the proper length of time for college. A graduate is spoken of as having "four years of college" even if it has taken him ten chronological years (part time) to acquire this education. A student who gets the required number of courses in less than four years is called "accelerated" (that is, faster than normal) and it is assumed that some extraordinary circumstance (such as large-scale warfare) must have prompted such a speed-up. When the Hutchins-sponsored University of Chicago college plan was put into operation, students explained to outsiders that their bachelor's degree was the equivalent of two years of college. The sponsors of the plan would certainly object to such a formulation, since they valued its uniqueness rather than its equivalence. But how else could the student explain to others just how far he had gone in college? And how else could he explain it to himself during those moments when he wanted to compare himself to the larger body of students in the United States?

In terms of the focus of interest in this book, the Cold War army and the educational system cases are, as a mathematician would say, trivial. They were presented only to approximate one end of a continuum of determinacy of career timetables. (The other end is much more difficult to point out.) All participants who reach the end have passed through the same stages—in the case of the army and the elementary and secondary school almost always in the same length of time, in the case of college in the same equivalent time units measured by semester hours' credit.

The division into smaller stages is useful to let any participant at any time know how far along he is and, as Uyeki puts it, to make the effort more "psychologically manageable." However, these bench marks are predetermined and agreed upon by everyone. There is nothing to be "doped out." There is no question about what subgroup of fellows to use as a model because they are all the same so far as their career timetable is concerned. There is, moreover, no room for bargaining on the timetable. A soldier's superior officer cannot shorten (or lengthen) the two-year stretch any more than the soldier can. Neither the professor nor the administrative officer of a college is in a position to reduce the number of credit hours needed for graduation, and, recognizing this, the students never demand that they do so. Of course, students *do* bargain with the faculty and the administration over other things—for example, schedules of classes, the amount of assigned work, course and examination grading, tuition and other charges. They may also bargain about credit hours when they argue that they should be passed rather than failed in a given course.

THE INDETERMINATE SENTENCE

A career timetable is removed from the trivial category as the details of its structure become indeterminate and uncertain. The experience of the indeterminate-sentence prisoner is perhaps a prototype of such a situation. In fact, a parallel can be drawn between such a prisoner and the TB patient, as shown in the accompanying statements.

Statement of an Indeterminate-Sentence Prisoner Whose Sentence Has Not Yet Been Set[9]

I was sentenced to San Quentin on an indefinite term. The prisoner there has no notion during the entire first year regarding the term the parole board will set for him to do. At the end of that year the parole board fixes his maximum, and may later reduce it. That first year is a perfect hell for a prisoner. He keeps asking others who were convicted of a similar offense about the details of their crime and of their maximum sentences. One man committed the same crime I did and he received a sentence of nine years but he had a long previous record and he was armed. Another man who was a first offender and who was not armed got four years. I was a first offender and was armed. Consequently I figure that I will get between four and nine years. But I keep thinking and worrying about it, for every year in prison makes a big difference. My worry is interfering with my work and I get sent to the "hole" for inefficiency in work. That looks bad on my record and I wonder whether it will increase my maximum sentence. This worry drives a person mad. As soon as the sentence is fixed, the prisoner can settle down to serve his time, and it is a great relief to have it settled.

---

9 E. H. Sutherland, *Principles of Criminology* (Philadelphia: J. B. Lippincott Co., 1947), pp. 527-28.

A Similar Statement as a Patient in a
Tuberculosis Hospital Might Tell It

I was sent to _____ Hospital for an indefinite term. The patient there has no notion when he first gets there regarding the term the medical board will set for him to do. When he finally gets boarded [has his case brought before a medical board for some kind of decision], he will find out when he is going to get surgery or get promoted to the exercise class. That first six to twelve months is a perfect hell for a patient. He keeps asking others who were hospitalized with a similar condition about the details of their disease and of the time they had to put in. One man had a cavity in one lung just as I do, and he spent twenty months in the hospital, but he had a long previous history of TB and could not take streptomycin. Another man had a fresh infection, took strep and INH, and stayed in the hospital twelve months. I was in for the first time, but was allergic to strep. Consequently, I figure that I will get between twelve and twenty months. But I keep thinking and worrying about it, for every month in the hospital makes a big difference. My worry is interfering with my treatment, and I get bawled out by the doctor because I'm up too much. That looks bad on my record and I wonder whether it will make the doctor refuse to give me a pass. This worry drives a person mad. As soon as a patient makes the exercise class or gets surgery, he can settle down to serve his last four to six months, and it is a great relief to have it settled.

An important property of the indeterminate sentence is the fact that no part of the timetable is given in advance. The prisoner, like the patient, is anxious to know what his sentence is, but he must "dope out" the clues to decide what his future is likely to be and what stage of progress he has reached. Timetable norms among prisoners develop, but they are not always followed in practice and the norms themselves are in a process of constant change.

Another important property of the indeterminate sentence is the fact that the participants can influence their timetable to some degree through control of their own behavior, which affects the reactions of others to them. The indeterminate-sentence prisoner does not start out with a set sentence like the draftee soldier, but can have some effect on his "set" by the way in which his records and his current behavior are evaluated by the parole board and the prison officials. The degree to which the timetable can currently be manipulated varies greatly from situation to situation. The prisoner cannot, for example, change his past record, which is one of the major factors used in setting the final sentence. The polio patient cannot affect the nerve damage that plays a major role in his rate of progress. In both cases, however, there is some leeway in the timetable bench marks that may be moved in one direction or the other as a result of the current behavior of the prisoner or patient.

The fact that the timetable may be influenced by current behavior means that there is room for bargaining. The prisoner or patient can make deals with his keepers or caretakers that will serve to shorten the stretch or bring the relaxation of restrictions at an earlier time. By "acting right" a more favorable decision may be won from the parole board or the medical board without overt demands. The fluidity of the timetable, while making the participant more anxious, also leaves some of the control in his hands.

The properties of the indeterminate sentence were clearly illustrated in the cases of the treatment of tuberculosis, polio, and mental disease. Before trying to make some general statements about career timetables, we might well take a brief look at several more career settings outside the field of medical treatment in which the reference points and end-points are more or less fluid and uncertain.

CHILD DEVELOPMENT

As an example of a less standardized timetable, we might take a look at child development. Here we find a plethora of bench marks, many of which have been carefully studied and catalogued. When does the infant first sit up, smile, reach for an object, crawl, walk, drink from a cup, say his first word, learn to control his bowels and bladder, use a spoon, etc.? As the child gets older, when does he learn to read various types of books, when can he shift from a tricycle to a bicycle, when does he learn to play certain games, when does he reach puberty, when does he become interested in the opposite sex, etc.? When *should* a concerted effort be made to toilet-train him? When *should* he be allowed to go outdoors alone, go away from home with groups of his own sex, have dates, borrow the car?

Parents discuss their children's progress with other parents. They compare the development of their child with that of other children and take note of the decisions other parents make about what their children may be allowed to or prompted to do. They are constantly trying to answer the question whether their child is developing as fast as he ought to—whether his rate of progress is normal or ab-normal. Bookish upper-middle-class parents may expand their uni-verse of comparison by reading the catalogues of Arnold Gesell; the less literary, by reading newspaper advice columns and articles in household magazines. The illiterate are limited to what they can see and hear among their circle of acquaintances.

The end-product—a mature, independent adult—is too remote a goal to be useful to a parent who wants to know how his child is getting along. The many reference points along the way serve as the markings on a measuring stick to let the parent know just how far the child has moved in the direction of adulthood in comparison with other children of his age. Such bench marks are more precise at some age periods than at others. Generally speaking, the reference points are much more clear-cut in infancy than in later childhood and adolescence. This difference has been increased in modern times by the rapid intergenerational changes in social expectations, which have affected the later childhood years much more than the early ones. The times of weaning and toilet-training have not been affected by social changes nearly as much as the times that a child is allowed to go away from home alone, have money of his own to spend, go on dates with the opposite sex. Such changes have not reached anything close to a new stable pattern, even within homogeneous social groups, and parents, like the Dover Sanatorium patients, do not know where they stand. Again like the Dover patients, such parents will grasp at any clue that looks as if it might show them the way out of their uncertainty, and they are consequently likely to follow clues that are not appropriate to their situation.

Parents do not simply compare their children to all other children, but most specifically to those social groups with whom they identify themselves. It is obvious that Americans have a different timetable of child development than, for example, the Arapesh or the Samoans. Within our own society it has often been pointed out that the expected times of weaning and toilet training are quite different for the middle and lower classes. A lower-class slum dweller who expects his children to contribute to the family income as soon as possible will be sharply critical of a son who has not made an effort to get a part-time job by the time he is twelve, while an upper-middle-class professional man who takes it for granted that his children will go to college considers a sixteen-year-old son's decision to follow a specific line of work as grossly premature. This difference in timetable expectations can be seen more clearly in the socially mobile family that must shift its expectations to fit the social group into which it is trying to move. The mother may be shocked at the idea of an eight-year-old girl going off to camp without her parents for several months until she learns that this is an accepted practice in the social group to which she aspires. When the child is upwardly mobile, but his parents are not, we have a clash in the timetables of the child and parents—a conflict that often is resolved by the child's cutting himself off more or less completely from his parents as soon as he is able to support himself ("going AMA," so to speak). Where a child is so severely physically or mentally disabled that he is not expected ever to reach independent adulthood, he is likely to be placed in an institution with others of his kind and is thus removed physically, as well as socially, from the promotion system.

Even without changes in social class levels, there is always some intergenerational conflict in timetables between children and parents as soon as children are old enough to think for themselves. The children, like their parents, come to think in terms of time-tables of their own development. They, too, want to know how they are progressing toward adulthood, when given restrictions on their freedom of behavior should be lifted, when given privileges should be extended to them. They, too, develop norms among their peers about when given stages should be reached. Such norms never agree completely with those of their parents and sometimes are in drastic conflict with them. Thus, the stage is set for bargaining over the timing of stages in social development.

For the most part, children (like TB patients) are pressing for earlier privileges, promotion in activity level, release from restrictions, and discharge from the treatment (parental direction). Parents (like the physicians) are trying to play safe by restricting activities and privileges until the disease (childhood) is brought under control. The parent, like the physician, is likely to trust the apparently co-operative child (patient) with privileges earlier than the one who does not seem to be able to take care of himself. Of course, some parents reject troublesome children in much the same way that a physician drives a troublemaker out of the hospital, and some "Momma's boys" cling to their parents right into adulthood in much the same way that an occasional patient finds a home in the hospital. But in both cases, this situation is regarded as abnormal by almost everyone concerned, and in both cases it receives a disproportionate share of attention from the experts on psychopathology.

A more thorough and detailed analysis of the timetable of child development would have to examine many more complexities of the situation than I have done here. For example, exactly what arguments, demands, and other bargaining techniques are used by each of the parties concerned in an effort to reach his goal, and what kinds of compromises are commonly worked out? The role and effectiveness of the common argument, "Everybody else is doing it," would be an especially interesting aspect for investigation. This argument by the underdog might be related to the controlling party's counter-argument, "If I let you do it, everybody will want to." Remember, too, that parents at one and the same time are the clients of teachers, advice columnists, and other child guidance experts and are authorities partially controlling the timetables of their children.

The developing child finds that he must bargain for his freedom with different people at different points in his career and under different circumstances. His parents are the main protagonists of his early years; later, teachers, youth leaders, and among some groups, the police, become important control agents. The boy who wants to extend his sexual experience in accordance with the expectations of his own sex peers first has to bargain with his parents for greater opportunity to make intimate contacts with girls (e.g., be allowed out late at night, get more spending money, borrow the family car), and must then bargain with the girls for the opportunity to engage in more advanced sexual activity. In fact, the latter kind of bargaining seems to follow an almost standardized sequence of stages from the initial date to sexual intercourse,[10] and if these stages were examined in terms of the scheme presented in this book, we might well find that a given social group had some norms (different for the boys and the girls) about how long each stage should take under given circumstances.

VERTICAL OCCUPATIONAL CAREERS

When we think of careers, we usually think of occupational careers. Until recent years, students of occupations concentrated most of their attention on the vertical career line—a career in which a person typically begins in a lowly position in an occupational or organizational structure and in time climbs a ladder of prestige,

[10] Winston Ehrmann, *Premarital Dating Behavior* (New York: Henry Holt and Co., 1959), p. 14.

authority, responsibility, and rewards, the rate and height of climb varying from person to person. A look at a few examples of such career lines will extend the concept of the career timetable.

The Business Executive

The career of the business executive in a corporation structure is one of the most frequently cited vertical career lines.[11] A man may begin in lower management (e.g., foreman) and work up into middle management. He may enter middle management directly from a university business school, a law school, or other specialized training and later move up to higher management (company policy-making level). Direct entry into higher management is unlikely except through family connections. Whatever the point of entry, the individual is seen as stepping on the rung of a ladder and the only proper direction of movement is up, except for brief horizontal excursions to other departments or locations for training and diversified experience.

One characteristic of the corporation management structure is its plethora of well-defined bench marks on the mobility ladder. Each position has a title that defines the occupant's authority and prestige relationships to others in his organization. A man can look back to see how long it took him to make each of the upward movements in the past. He can observe the experience of those who are ahead of him and listen to their stories to get an idea of how long it should take him to make the next movement ahead. In a stable organization with a stable timetable, the expected rate of advancement can be judged quite precisely.

[11] The term "business executive" includes a rather wide diversity of career patterns. The illustrations used here pertain most directly to the production departments of a manufacturing company at the lower and middle management levels. Recruitment becomes more complex at the higher management level because many—probably most—of those selected come from sales and finance rather than production. A thorough company-wide study of career timetables would, of course, have to take these converging lines of promotion into consideration.

The executive can learn what the signs of promotion or coming promotion are. If it is common practice at a given level of middle management to shift the executives to three or four different departments for about six months each for diversified experience, he may assume that he is on his way to promotion once he is being put through such a routine of transfers. However, if he is shifted to another department and left for more than a year, he may have reason to wonder whether he has been passed over and will be left in this position. The significance of horizontal shifts varies at different points in the hierarchy. Martin and Strauss[12] report on one company in which horizontal movement at the lower management level indicates unsatisfactory performance. At middle management levels it indicates training and testing for higher management, and *lack of horizontal movement* indicates unsatisfactory performance. In higher management, there is again very little horizontal movement.

Corporation management is quite age-conscious, and within a given business norms will develop about how old candidates for given positions should be. A promotion may be refused on the grounds that the candidate is too old. If he does not move out of a certain position by a certain age, he is likely to remain there. Such age norms enable the candidates themselves to judge their chances of further promotion. "A person who does not progress in accordance with these age timetables may know, therefore, that his potential for higher levels of management has been judged unfavorably."[13] Thus, in one company, a man beginning at the foreman level is expected to be ready for middle management by age 35, seasoned between ages 30 and 40, and moved up to higher management by age 40, or at latest 45. If a man is nearing the age at which he will be too old for promotion in a given company, he may well consider the possibility of taking a job with a different company

[12] Norman H. Martin and Anselm L. Strauss, "Patterns of Mobility within Industrial Organizations," *Journal of Business*, 29 (1956), 101-10. The illustrations and ideas in this section are taken in large part from this paper.

[13] Martin and Strauss, p. 103.

whose structure and career norms offer a better chance of promotion at this age. Of course, such decision-making presupposes that the executive accumulates information about the promotion system, not only of his own company, but of others that he might regard as alternative employers. We may expect that a common subject of gossip among corporation executives from different companies is concerned with the details of career contingencies at their various places of work, though, so far as I am aware, this aspect of the business world has not been carefully studied.

An important point made by Martin and Strauss is that certain positions are *testing points* that determine what direction a career line will take. In one auto parts industry the position of general foreman in a production unit is a testing point to determine whether the individual should be moved up to middle management. In the middle management range, a major testing point is assistant division manager. Higher management observes the individual in this position and decides whether he is competent to be put in line for higher executive positions. If not, he is likely to be promoted to the next higher position and left there.

The positions that are testing points from the viewpoint of higher management are viewed by the individual candidate as critical junctures where he faces a number of alternative directions, some of which are dead ends (but may be secure positions of high specialization). He must judge the next moves that he is involved in to decide what they mean in terms of his career. Is he being left in a given position too long? Is the move to a somewhat higher position at a branch factory a step in the promotion system or exile to Siberia? Is a move to a staff position a means of utilizing his special skills, or is he being sidetracked from the production line promotion system? On the basis of such interpretations, a man judges where he stands, what he can expect in the future, and what he might be able to do to influence his timetable. For example, pressure on his superiors may speed up his timetable of promotion, but it may also cause him to be more quickly and definitely rejected. The ambitious executive must take care to compare himself to appropriate career models. If he believes he has been placed in a given position in a given department only as a temporary training assignment, he cannot compare himself to others for whom the same position means the end of the line of promotion.

The Airline Pilot

The career bench marks and testing points of the airline pilot were the subject of a study by L. Wesley Wager.[14] Some of these career contingency points, as Wager calls them, are administratively standardized and come at regular intervals—for example, the monthly reports on copilots and the quarterly flight checks for captains. Some are an inevitable part of the career but not so precisely timed—transition schools, upgrading schools, change from flying reserve to a regular schedule. In such cases, the pilot—like the hospital patient or business executive—is faced with the task of trying to figure out when each of these points in his career should be attained and what it means when a given point is reached much earlier or much later than expected. Finally, there are the contingency points that are rare and unexpected (except perhaps in an actuarial sense) and therefore cannot be anticipated and planned for—the "technical emergencies" and "irregularities." The way in which a pilot handles an emergency or the nature and seriousness of an irregularity for which he is responsible is evaluated by his superiors (if they know about it) and may be entered into his company record and thus affect future assignments and promotion, or, in a serious case, cause him to be suspended or discharged.

As in the case of the business executive, the company conceives of some of the contingency points as testing points. The transition schools, where the pilot is trained and tested in a type of aircraft that he has not yet flown, are used this way, especially for the junior copilot. Every pilot is expected eventually to become a

[14] "Career Patterns and Role Problems of Airline Pilots in a Major Airline Company," Ph.D. dissertation, Department of Sociology, University of Chicago, 1959. [I have added my own interpretation to some of Wager's information.]

captain capable of flying all the different kinds of aircraft used by the company. If, therefore, he is unable to master satisfactorily the control of any type of aircraft, he has no future with the company and may be discharged. The transition school is especially crucial for the first-year probationary pilot, who may be discharged by the company for any cause and is likely to be dropped after any failure without being given another chance.

There are important differences, however, between the ways in which the testing points are used for business executives and for pilots. In the case of the executive, it is usually not a question of complete success with promotion or complete failure with discharge. The executive who does not win the confidence of his superiors may be "cooled out" in various ways, even being promoted another step before being shelved in a fairly high-level, but dead-end, position. He may be transferred to a less important location, given a noncrucial staff position, given a raise and higher-sounding title without corresponding authority or responsibility—but he is still a business executive even though no longer moving up the ladder. The career of the pilot does not offer these alternatives. The pilot *must* keep moving up the ladder until he eventually becomes a senior captain—or flunk out along the way and cease to be a pilot. Airline piloting apparently has no chronic sidetrack for the unwanted. It is a matter of "up or out," with no euphemisms to protect the failures.

This is not to say that the pilot has no control whatever over his career timetable. Wager points out a number of ways in which a pilot may slow down or speed up certain career phases. He can put off transition schools or upgrading schools for a time by claiming that he is not ready. (However, he cannot stall such school assignments very long and he must always consider whether his temporary refusal makes a poor impression on his superiors.) The copilot can make himself ready for upgrading more quickly by getting himself assigned to captains who are more generous in giving their copilot an opportunity to fly the plane. He can select a domicile (home airport) that has relatively few pilots with higher seniority and therefore a better chance for faster promotion (or do just the opposite if he feels unready for upgrading). He may control the adverse effect that irregularities may have on his career timetable by covering up the irregularities whenever possible.[15]

In order to exercise such control, however, the pilot needs information. If he wants to manipulate domicile assignments, he must know what the seniority lists for the various domiciles are, what their schedule of operations is, how the local managers handle requests for changing the schedule of schools and captain-copilot assignments, and so on. To decide whether or not he should try to delay a given transitional school, the pilot must know what kind of performance the school requires, whether it will be held against him if he has insufficient practice, what will happen if he does not pass the test the first time, and so on. In fact, pilots are *not* well informed on such matters. They are not, like the hospital patient, surrounded by sources of information. Their work schedules are such that they see very little of their colleagues—especially those colleagues who are closest to them in their career timetable. They are largely removed from the scene of operations about which they must make predictions, again unlike the TB patient who learns much about his own future by just keeping his eyes and ears open. The junior copilot, who has the greatest need for such information, usually has the least access to it. Wager points out that an important function of the transitional schools is to bring together groups of pilots at about the same career stage in one place for a number of weeks where they can spend some time in informal exchange of information about the planes, the company, the captains, the flight managers, the domiciles, the rules and their evasion, and the other conditions of work, and thus return to their job somewhat better equipped to predict and control their career.

The change in the career timetable norms, which has occurred in TB treatment as a result of changes in treatment methods, can be illustrated even more dramatically in the airline pilot's career. Be-

15 Wager points out that it is a general belief among pilots that irregularities will be interpreted against the pilot by airline officials even when there is good evidence that the pilot was not at fault, and, therefore, pilots tend to say as little as possible in their flight reports and especially to keep details about rule violations, irregularities, and emergencies to a minimum.

cause of rapid changes in the size and nature of the airline industry, the changes in rules controlling aircraft operations, and the repeated introduction of new types of aircraft, the timetable of career phases has undergone some marked shifts through the years. Wager dealt directly with this issue by dividing his pilot subjects into groups which started their airline careers before 1939, 1939-44, 1945-49, and after 1949 and collecting information on such matters as how long they were copilots on reserve, captains on reserve, and copilots before upgrading, and how much time elapsed between transitional schools. The interested reader may find the details in Wager's dissertation. It is sufficient here to note that the earlier phases of the career are being stretched out. Thus, the pilots starting with the company in the 1950's take longer on the average to make captain than those who started in the 1930's. Almost all the other career phases have been lengthened in the same way. For example, while the majority of those starting with the company in the 1930's was flying a regular monthly schedule in less than a year after being upgraded, those starting with the company in the late 1940's in almost all cases needed more than three years after upgrading to achieve such a schedule.

Wager did not deal directly with the actual process of developing timetable norms and using them for predicting and controlling one's own timetable. However, we may speculate about the effect that the stretching out of contingency points and the paucity of information about career contingencies may have on prediction and control. The new junior copilot has the greatest opportunity for collecting information about the career timetable from the captains with whom he flies, but the experience of these captains, who started five to twenty years earlier, may be quite inappropriate to his own case. When he hears these captains tell of being upgraded in less than two years and flying a regular schedule shortly after, the new-generation pilot may wonder what is wrong when he is still flying copilot four years later. He may even wonder whether this is a reflection on his own competence. And what does the older captain think of these younger men who still have not been upgraded three, four, or five years after beginning their airline careers?

If the matter were simply a contrast between the twenty-year men and the newcomers, the timetable changes would be readily recognized and corrections made. However, when you have all the intermediate groups with progressive changes throughout the years, it may be difficult for a group at any particular point to know what expectations are reasonable for *them*. Under such circumstances it is probably difficult to develop stable norms of a career timetable. I suspect that the newer pilots—insofar as they are able to obtain relevant information—tend to use the group just a little ahead of them as a reference group to develop their own norms. If so, they are likely to believe that their own timetable is lagging behind the norm.

THE "WORKING CLASS" CAREER

It is not true, as the bias of sociological studies of occupations might lead us to believe, that most occupational careers operate through a vertical mobility system. Even in the professions there are some well established, institutionalized patterns of horizontal mobility. The urban public school teacher—especially a woman—seldom moves up a hierarchy, but instead moves from a "poor" school—usually in the slums where most of the openings for new teachers are—to "better" schools in middle-class neighborhoods with more teachable and controllable children and parents.[16]

Among employed persons as a whole, the "orderly career"—either vertical or horizontal—is perhaps the exception rather than the rule. A large proportion of people moves frequently, not only from one job to another, but also from one line of work to another in a sequence that does not fit into a related progression of jobs.[17] Even in such cases, however, the concept of a career timetable may be applicable because each unrelated segment of such a "disorderly"

[16] Howard S. Becker, "The Career of the Chicago Public Schoolteacher," *American Journal of Sociology*, 57 (March, 1952), 470-77.

[17] Harold Wilensky, "Orderly Careers and Social Participation," *American Sociological Review*, 26 (August, 1961), 521-39.

work career may be more or less structured in terms of an expected sequence and approximate timing of stages or events.

Semi-skilled factory workers at first sight seem to be a rather static group. They do much the same kind of work year after year and never move up an occupational ladder. Upon closer examination, however, we find that even within a given factory there is a great deal of moving around from job to job. This movement is by no means haphazard, but follows rather clear-cut patterns. As far as I am aware, the timetables of such movements have not been specifically investigated, but some studies of production workers in auto assembly plants provide hints about how such a timetable may operate.[18]

There is *some* upward movement to the lower grade of supervision among auto workers. It is usually assumed that they have little chance of making the grade if they have not been promoted to foreman by the age of forty. Before that time, they have to make a step in the direction of foremanship by moving a step higher in the wage labor scale—group worker, skilled workman. Supervision, however, is not the goal of most of the workers. "Unlike the professional or the salaried office-holder, the factory worker does not see his present job as part of a career pattern which channels his aspirations and sustains his hope."[19]

But the workers *do* rate the wage labor jobs for which they are eligible and seek to transfer to jobs that are less demanding, have less supervision, are cleaner, have fewer layoffs, are less monotonous. They move from line-tender to line repairman, from the assembly line to machine operation, from production jobs to inspection and service. Such transfers depend mainly on seniority and on information about job openings gleaned through informal communication channels. The main assembly line is almost always the least popular job and therefore that to which the new unskilled workman is likely

[18] I have drawn upon the following works in this section: Charles R. Walker and Robert H. Guest, *The Man on the Assembly Line* (Cambridge, Mass.: Harvard University Press, 1952); Ely Chinoy, *Automobile Workers and the American Dream* (New York: Doubleday and Company, Inc., 1955).

[19] Chinoy, p. 117.

to be assigned. As he gets to know the ropes, he begins to angle for openings on subassembly lines, bench jobs, repair work, and so on.

Individual workers who intend to stay with the company for a time must try to estimate how long it will take them to get off the assembly line, how long it will take to transfer from machine operation to a nonproduction job. The workers discuss their experiences and expectations about how long such moves "should" take and thereby develop a measuring stick by which each worker can tell whether or not he is behind schedule. Perhaps, too, the threat of falling behind schedule causes the worker to apply pressure on the personnel department, supervisors, and union representatives in much the same way that the TB patient applies pressure on the physician for faster promotions when he is not moving toward discharge as fast as he "should." Such timetables on the part of the auto workers may be very unstable and often "unrealistic" when they fail to keep up with the economic ups and downs of the industry. For example, transfer into "better" jobs could be had more quickly during a period of rapid expansion, such as the Korean War, and more slowly during slack periods, such as 1957-58. However, the behavior of the Dover TB patients shows that unreliability of the clues does not stop people from trying to construct a timetable from which they can make predictions about their future.[20]

The Worker Off the Job

The job is not expected to have any intrinsic attraction for the auto worker as it is supposed to for the research scientist, the professor, the skilled craftsman, the executive. A "better" job is one

[20] Chinoy in a personal communication suggests that the conceptions of time perspectives that I have used to explain some of the behavior of auto workers may have to be modified for the social class and cultural differences in time perspectives between the social background usually found among auto workers and that found among business executives or professional workers following a vertical career. A clarification of this issue requires studies more directly focused on a comparison of definitions of time among different social groups in our society. I *can* say that in the TB hospital, the differences in social class origin of the patients did not seem to make any difference in the manner in which they developed or used treatment timetable norms.

that slightly increases his income or job security or conserves his energy so that he will be better able to use his off-work time. As David Riesman puts it in his introduction to Chinoy's book, ". . . success at one's job may increasingly be thought less important than 'success' in one's general style of life, at home and off the job."[21]

Perhaps it is of less consequence to the worker when he will get off the assembly line than when he can get a new car, a new set of furniture, a new refrigerator, a home of his own, or pay off the mortgage. (Chinoy found that workers often defined "getting ahead" as the accumulation of possessions.) Here he will compare himself to his neighborhood or acquaintanceship group rather than to his fellow workers (though the two may overlap). Within such groups, we could—upon close and detailed examination—very likely find expectations about how long one "should" have to save to buy a home, how often to trade in the car, when and how often to have children, and so on. Such collective "keeping up with the Joneses" is not simply a product of each person or family's trying to match the social prestige of neighbors and acquaintances. It is also a way of establishing reference points on a consumption timetable so that the individual (or family) will have a way of telling whether he is moving toward his goals as a consumer at a reasonable pace, whether he is getting there too slowly, or whether he is doing so well that he is progressing much faster than generally expected. After all, such concepts as "reasonable," "average," "slow," and "fast" have meaning only in comparison to some standard. The time-table norms of a group in relation to the goals of its members provide the members with such a standard against which they can evaluate their progress and thus, to some degree, escape from the uncertainty of not knowing where they stand.

[21] Chinoy, p. xi.

5

The Study of the Career Timetables

People will not accept uncertainty. They will make an effort to structure it no matter how poor the materials they have to work with and no matter how much the experts try to discourage them.

One way to structure uncertainty is to structure the time period through which uncertain events occur. Such a structure must usually be developed from information gained from the experience of others who have gone or are going through the same series of events. As a result of such comparisons, norms develop for entire groups about when certain events may be expected to occur. When many people go through the same series of events, we speak of this as a career and of the sequence and timing of events as their career timetable.

The illustrations of career timetables that I have used in this book are for the most part ones that were selected *because* they were relatively easy to analyze and present to the reader. They were ones on which relatively detailed information was available and on which the career timetable was most clearly structured. I have briefly speculated on a few areas where a timetable structure is not at all clear-cut—for example, horizontal movements in occupational careers and consumption timetables. In these cases there is insufficient information available to make an analysis of a career sequence, and we cannot even be sure they fit the criteria of career timetables used in this book. For example, there has been considerable study of consumption patterns in relation to the life cycle, especially the family life cycle, but such studies have been almost entirely of the gross statistical relationship type—that is, what quantity of given products or services is purchased at given stages of the life cycle. There has been virtually no study of the process of decisions and actions of consumer purchase of given families over an extended period of time. But it is this type of study that is needed if a timetable of consumership with its many complexities and interrelationships is to be revealed.

I contend that it may be worthwhile to study career timetables in a variety of areas (in most cases probably as part of a broader study of a career), including areas where a timetable structure now seems obscure. In this chapter I review the dimensions and issues of such a study, note some cautions and qualifications that one might watch for, and make a tentative effort to point out the definitions and boundaries of career timetables.

CONDITIONS FOR TIMETABLE NORMS

From an examination of the careers illustrated in this book, the following conditions appear to be necessary for timetables to develop:

1. The series of events or conditions under scrutiny must be thought of in terms of a career—a series of related and definable stages or phases of a given sphere of activity that a group of people goes through in a progressive fashion (that is, one step leads to another) in a given direction or on the way to a more or less definite and recognizable end-point or goal or series of goals. This means that there must be a group definition of success or attainment of a goal. Such definitions may be provided by movement through an institutional hierarchy (business executive careers, academic careers); through a series of contingencies moving in a given direction

(the private practice physician getting a better clientele, better office location, better hospital appointments; the schoolteacher getting better school assignments or more desirable courses to teach); escape from an undesirable situation (the patient getting out of a hospital, the prisoner getting out of jail, the draftee getting out of the army); or development in a given direction (children developing toward independent adulthood).

2. There must be an interacting (not necessarily face-to-face) group of people with access to the same body of clues for constructing the norms of a timetable.

A CULTURE-BOUND PHENOMENON

Anthropologists, in their reports on primitive groups, have in many cases pointed out that the concept of time of the people they studied is quite different from our own. Although ideas about the nature and structuring of time are quite diverse, they seem to fall into two main patterns:

> Epochal time . . . may be seen as a vast continuum of progress and catastrophe or it may be interpreted as a great cyclic system featuring the restoration of virtue to government after each inevitable fall, as in the Chinese sense of history. The metaphors commonly used by speakers of English—the stream of time, Father Time, the pressure of time—are not those of other languages, and time often is not personified at all. Time may be relatively so unimportant to a people that their sense of history does not even include knowing one's own age. On the other hand, it may dominate a people's thought to such an extent that the measurement of time may become a preoccupation. To such a society, time is a commodity to be spent, lost, invested, saved, wasted, thrown away, or employed to best advantage. Its passage is marked in terms of very fine distinctions and past time is studded with memorial days, anniversaries, and foundings.[1]

[1] Robert J. Smith, "Cultural Differences in the Life Cycle and the Concept of Time," in *Aging and Leisure*, ed. Robert W. Kleemeier (New York: Oxford University Press, 1961), p. 85.

These two orientations toward time are dealt with specifically in Murray Wax's comparison of the world view and time perspectives of the Pawnee Indians and the Bible-era Hebrews.[2]

In his analysis of Pawnee mythology and way of life Wax notes the lack of attention to accurate measures of time. Often the Pawnees do not even keep track of the calendar month. Life is seen as a series of repetitions or cycles—day and night, one season to another and return, misfortune and blessing, poverty and wealth. They search for turning points, for example, for a movement from a condition of being hungry, cold, wet, and poor to being sated, warm, dry, and rich. But such a change is not a progression; it merely turns attention to an expectation of a change back to the former condition. There is no need to plan for the future—good fortune is not the culmination of planning and labor, but the consequence of a blessed relationship with the supernatural.

The examination of the writings of the Hebrews of the Biblical era shows the development of a quite different time perspective. The Old Testament, according to Wax, is written with "a linear sense of history—a conception of time as the dimension along which action moves simply and straightforwardly, in an immutable sequence of cause and effect."[3] The religion did not celebrate the birth and death and rebirth of the gods with the passage of the seasons as the religions of agricultural societies often do. Yahweh never died. He was not the god of the yearly round, but of crucial events, and his rewards and punishments could be extended into the future. In the Old Testament, history is progress. One version of this history even has a clear-cut final goal—the coming of the Kingdom of God— and the events along the way may be regarded as bench marks of progress.[4]

---

[2] Murray Wax, "Time, Magic and Asceticism: A Comparative Study of Time Perspectives," Ph.D. dissertation, Department of Sociology, University of Chicago, 1959, especially Chaps. 3, 6, 8, 9.

[3] *Ibid.*, p. 79.

[4] Although I do not want to become involved in a discussion of the reasons for the development of such a time perspective, I note only that Wax suggests

Wax names the Pawnee-type view the "closed time system" and the Biblical Hebrew view the "open time system." The closed time system seems to be found in most primitive cultures and in many of the older civilizations that do not stem from the ancient Hebrew. The open time system became part of the cultural heritage that passed from ancient Judaism to early Christianity and has come to dominate the more "advanced" parts of the present-day world.

In the closed system people do not know their ages in years, but deduce their ages from their development. In the open system, development is thought of as time-serving—so many years of age, school, etc. In the closed system work is regulated by conditions—weather, hunger—and one rests when he is supplied with his needs or when the weather prevents work. In the open system work and leisure are regulated by the clock and calendar.

It is obvious that my definitions of careers and the conditions under which timetable norms develop correspond to Wax's open time system. This same time perspective is implicit throughout my discussion of the timetable of tuberculosis treatment and the structuring of time in my other examples. In fact, the structuring of events into a career can occur *only* when one thinks in terms of such an open time system. The career timetable with its attendant phenomena is, therefore, a culture-bound concept.

It is, however, a culture-bound concept whose area of application is apparently spreading and becoming more pronounced. In our society the segment of the population that tends to adhere to the open time system in its more extreme form is the professional and executive middle class, and this is precisely the segment that is increasing proportionately in the total population and whose values dominate our major institutions. The English language, which expresses the open time system more explicitly than any other major

---

that the Hebrew view was the reaction of an underdog society surrounded by powerful neighbors, a reaction designed to convince the Hebrews that they would be successful and obtain progressively greater success (though there might be temporary setbacks) because the deity had so planned it.

language, is spreading rapidly throughout the world as a second language and in many areas as the first language of the educated class. The Communist world has long been dominated by the concept of a timetable of progress, a timetable of winning out over capitalism. In fact, Communism as a political and philosophical ideology has perhaps carried the idea of a historical march of events toward an inevitable goal to the most extreme form in which it has yet appeared. The newly independent "underdeveloped" nations are concerned with "catching up" with the more economically advanced nations. The plans for social and economic improvement that they have been issuing in recent years are essentially timetables of the catching-up process. The populations in which the closed time system holds sway grow steadily smaller.

Allowing, then, for such a cultural limitation, what issues must be considered in the study of a career timetable? In the remainder of this chapter I deal with those issues which had an important place in the analysis of the tuberculosis treatment career and the other careers that served as illustrations in this book. Of course, further study may considerably add to and modify this scheme of analysis.

SPLITTING UP BLOCKS OF TIME

Everyone, even the back ward mental hospital patient, makes use of various devices to break up the days, weeks, months, and years of his life into smaller units. Such division of large masses into smaller blocks occurs not only in relation to time. We divide books into chapters, chapters into sections, sections into subsections and paragraphs. We divide academic disciplines into specialty areas, topics, and courses so that the subject matter may be viewed a little at a time. When a long series of digits must be memorized, people invariably break the series up into groups of a few digits each and memorize the digits in these groups rather than as an undifferentiated series of digits. These examples are perhaps all different aspects of the same psychological phenomenon.

However, although the splitting of time periods into smaller units probably always goes with the development of timetable norms, this process in itself does not make a career timetable. The units into which the chronic patient breaks up his days and weeks show no discernible direction or movement toward discharge from the hospital or other goal. The life prisoner can look forward to Sunday as a welcome break in a dreary routine, but the succession of Sundays does not lead him anywhere. The division of time into units with recurring markers may make one's life more psychologically manageable, but it does not in itself make a career timetable. For such a timetable to develop, the reference points must move in some definable direction or toward some recognizable goal.

THE MEANING OF REFERENCE POINTS

In all timetables we find dividing points for events that serve as signposts for progress in a given direction (toward discharge or graduation or adulthood, attaining family security or racial equality or a certain occupational position). In retrospect, such signposts may also serve as reference points from which one may predict and measure further progress.

Reference points may be more or less clear-cut and stable. If they are prescribed in detail and rigidly adhered to, as in the career of pupils in our school system, one's movement through the timetable is almost completely predictable. As the reference points become less rigid and less clear-cut, they must be discovered and interpreted through observation and through interaction with others of one's career group. The more unclear the reference points are, the harder it is for members of a career group to know where they stand in relation to others and the more likely it is that they will attend to inappropriate clues and thus make grossly inaccurate predictions concerning future progress. The degree of stability is related in part to the changes in timetables through time. Such changes may be gradual and almost imperceptible or they may occur quickly, as in military careers in time of war, occupational careers during economic expansion or depression, and disease careers at a time of drastic changes in treatment methods.

The meanings of such reference points are learned by members of the group through observation of the experience of other members and through the communication of experiences, ideals, myths, and hopes among the members of the group. During a time of rapid change in the timetable when the changes are not made explicit, such information will contain many contradictions and thus make the construction of stable and reliable timetable norms more difficult. We may conceive of an extreme situation where rapidity of change and lack of explicit information may make the development of group timetable norms impossible. Not that members of the group will not keep trying, but that their judgments will so often be so far wrong that they lose confidence in their ability to make predictions of their future. None of the careers we have used as illustrations approaches this extreme, and it is difficult to invent a realistic group traversing the same career line without some fairly accurate norms of progress. In any case, the stability of norms is relative. They are more stable (and more accurately predictive) for Valentine Hospital TB patients than for Dover Sanatorium patients, for railroad firemen and engineers than for airline pilots; but in no case do they seem to be completely absent.[5]

---

[5] Where we have professional-client or boss-subordinate relationships, it is not only the underdog, but also his superior, who is confused by sharp changes in timetable contingencies. When treatment methods undergo a sudden shift, not only do the patients have greater difficulty anticipating their future careers, but the physicians also become much more doubtful about when patients should be given privileges or be discharged—until a new set of norms to accompany the new treatment has been worked out. When a corporation is drastically reorganized, not only is the junior executive's timetable thrown into temporary confusion, but his bosses also have much greater difficulty deciding when their subordinates are "ready" for promotion under the new circumstances.

When career contingencies change as a result of adding alternative career lines to an existing traditional career structure, the problem of estimating norms is often dealt with by equating the reference points for the new lines to the old ones. A good example is the present-day development of academic and quasi-academic careers. The traditional career signposts have been blurred in recent years by the enormous increase in university nonfaculty research appointments and the employment of academic research people by industry, foundations, and government agencies. The pressure of researchers to know where they stand in relation to their fellows has often been met by making their positions equivalent to positions in the traditional system. The industrial research organization imitates the university graduate department in its table of organization (while borrowing the labels from business); heads of government research agencies informally equate a given GS rank to an academic rank; the university research associate becomes "research associate (assistant professor)."

The reference points and stages of a timetable do *not* necessarily describe what a person is actually doing at a given stage of the timetable, but serve only as symbols of such activity. A "bed rest" patient who is promoted to an "exercise" classification may already have been as active as an exercise patient is supposed to be while he was still on bed rest. The promotion is important in letting him know where he stands on the road to discharge even though it tells us nothing at all about the amount of activity that this patient engaged in before or after his promotion. With the slow promotions in the peacetime army, it is not unusual for a captain, let us say, to carry out the tasks that the table of organization prescribes for a major for a long period of time before he is actually promoted to major. The promotion is an extremely important point in his career—especially for a regular army officer—even though it may not make the slightest difference in the work that he performs. It is important to study just how close the formal definitions of timetable reference points or stages are to the actual activity of the participants at those points or stages. The greater the discrepancy between the two, the greater will be the discrepancy between status and function in that particular career line and the more "unrealistic" will be the status distinctions.

THE SEARCH FOR A REFERENCE GROUP

Career lines may be divided between those where each participant starts running as soon as he comes to the track (continuous system) and those where the participants have to wait for a bunch to collect before starting off (cohort system).[6] Of the illustrations used in this book, only the draftee army and the school system use a cohort system. With this system there can be no doubt what the appropriate reference group is for measuring one's progress—one starts off and travels with the same group all the way.

With a continuous belt, on the other hand, it is not so clear who one's closest colleagues are. Not only does each begin at a different time, but each moves ahead at a different rate. The participant must not only "dope out" the nature and sequence of the bench marks; he must also construct an appropriate subgroup from among his potential colleagues to serve as a primary model for his own career expectations or hopes—a model group that contains at least some members who are slightly ahead of him in the timetable so that he may use their experience to anticipate his own future. Thus, parents compare the development of their children mainly with that of others in the social circle with which they identify. TB patients compare themselves primarily with other patients receiving the same type of treatment and having the same kind of disease condition so far as the patients can tell. The academic man compares himself with others aiming for the same type of institution. Business executives compare themselves primarily with colleagues with similar ambitions working in the same type of organization.

[6] Erving Goffman called my attention to this distinction.

The way in which the member of a career group decides which subgroup to identify himself with for timetable purposes might be thought of as the sociological side of what psychologists call "level of aspiration." A person attaches himself to a faster or a slower moving subgroup depending upon what set of expectations he thinks he can meet.

Not everyone climbs on a given career belt and sticks to it. Changing career belts is common in our society—perhaps far more common than our bias for studying conceptually static situations would lead us to believe. The patient may recognize that his condition is markedly better or worse than he first thought or that his treatment program has been drastically altered; and, therefore, he seeks new models to help predict a newly conceived future. A physician may start out his career as a general practitioner and later decide to restrict his practice to a specialty, or—as is increasingly becoming necessary in order to make such a shift—to take off a period of time for the training and supervised work required for entering a specialty. A family may move for a time in line with the expectations of a given social class and then decide to set its sights on moving into a higher stratum. The factory worker whose primary job interest was union politics may decide that he would rather try for a supervisory position with the company.

Whenever such a career shift is made, the participant must figure out a new timetable with new reference points. The old one, if not shucked off, may only lead him astray. The academic man who has succeeded in making a shift from a small teachers college to a major university must take on a new set of expectations including some important differences in his career timetable norms. The issues are no longer such things as the time when he gets a chance at summer and evening teaching, is able to determine class schedules, or obtains a foothold in the administrative hierarchy, but rather the timing of publications, research projects, and the right to organize seminars for select students. His models are no longer fellow college faculty members, but a nationwide professional colleague group from similar institutions. Unless the person can shift his career norms to fit the new setting, his predictions of his career timetable will not be useful to him.

Of course, the academic man making such a shift is likely to have prepared himself for it in advance. In many career areas, however, such preparation is less likely to occur. Students of social mobility, for example, have noted that people attempting to switch their identification to a higher social class often do so with great naïveté and make mistakes in their timing of given kinds of interaction with others that reduce the chances of their being accepted into the status to which they aspire. Important dimensions in the study of career timetables, therefore, are the readiness or the difficulty with which a given shift in a career may be accomplished and the characteristics of careers that make such shifts more or less difficult.

SHIFTING TIME PERSPECTIVES

Another aspect of a career timetable that deserves attention is the change that may occur in timetable perspectives during the course of the career. We have seen in the case of the long-term hospital patient how the timetable norms lengthen with increasing duration of hospitalization, at least up to a certain point. The patient frequently starts out identifying himself with those who are in for a short time. Only after he himself has passed this stage does he begin to think of himself as staying the "average" time, and then he even advances the average somewhat when he stays longer until it becomes obvious that he is being kept "overtime."

We may wonder whether the same process occurs in other careers. The new executive trainee fresh out of college fancies himself, let us say, a department head by age 30 and revises this expectation upward only when he reaches age 30 without being near this goal. The average, he finds from observation, seems to be between ages 35 and 40, so he still has plenty of time. When he has not reached this level by age 40, he may note that in a number of cases other men did not reach the department-head level until age 45, so he still has a chance. Only when he is approaching age 50 without making the grade does he finally admit that he is clearly behind schedule.

Do such shifts in perspectives occur in occupational groups, with parents observing and directing their children's development, with families trying to keep pace with the social and economic advancement of their social circle, or on the part of politicians striving to work their way up through a hierarchy of public offices? And what is the attitude toward those who are very far ahead or very far behind the timetable norms? Do such attitudes have the effect of moving the actual careers of individuals closer to the group norms as they do in the case of tuberculosis and polio patients?

Shifting perspectives are probably more common in some types of careers than in others. We may expect a lag in the norms when a career timetable is changing rapidly, as with the airline pilots whose career stages are being slowed up or with middle-class children whose developmental timetable is being speeded up. Perhaps a lack of explicitness in timetable bench marks also makes such shifting of perspectives during the course of one's career more likely.

HANDLING FAILURE

A career timetable is, as I mentioned earlier, a tight production schedule which not all those following the career path can keep up with. Some fall so far behind and have so little chance of catching up—either in the reasonably near future, or ever—that the normal timetable no longer applies to them except to show how much they have fallen by the wayside.

The proportion of such "failures" varies widely from one career line to another. In some—for example, public school pupils—it is a small proportion of the total; in others—for example, nursing home inmates—it is a majority. In some cases the definition of failure is sharp and unmistakable and is symbolized by shifting the person to a different social and/or geographical location—for example, the patient moved from an intensive treatment unit to a chronic service. In other cases, failure to keep up to the mark in the promotion system is never clearly established, and there is an accumulation of borderline cases who may or may not be considered failures depending upon slight differences of interpretation of their career experiences—for example, business executive careers, where it is often not clear whether many of the men in intermediate positions have been left behind or are still in the running, but on the slow side of the norm.

There must be some provision in every career line for those who cannot keep up to the mark, especially those who are being left hopelessly behind to the point where they become a class apart. In some career lines, the failures may be uncompromisingly shucked off —airline piloting seems to approach this extreme. In other career lines, however, the total society or some organized part of it has made a commitment to a given category of its members that cannot easily be rejected. Care and treatment of the ill and education of the young are typical of such career lines in the United States. Those who cannot possibly approach the normal timetable of recovery or learning must still be cared for, but in a different way and with a different set of expectations. A "chronic sidetrack" is created for them. They are still pupils, but in an ungraded class or a special school. They are still patients, but receiving largely maintenance care rather than active treatment. They are still part of the domain occupied by their career group, but no longer part of the forward-moving promotion system.

There are intermediate ways of dealing with timetable failures. In many universities and in large, well-established businesses there is often an obligation to provide a job for the professor or executive even when he is no longer considered useful to the organization. Because of the nature of the relationship, the unwanted incumbents cannot be moved off to a dead-end sidetrack in as blatant a manner as can the public hospital patient or the public school pupil who is considered hopeless. (However, systems of compulsory retirement with loopholes for excepting individuals who are still wanted sometimes operate as such a sidetrack at the upper age range.) The sidetracking in such cases must operate more subtly, often with the notion of failure or rejection denied or obscured by a consolation prize.

An important issue to investigate, then, in any study of a career timetable is the manner in which failure is handled, both by those who suffer the failure and by others who play a part in the control of their career timetables. When a number of studies dealing with this issue has been made, we may be able to specify in more detail the conditions under which different modes of handling failure are applied. For example, does a firm commitment by a public agency to provide long-term service to a given category of people invariably lead to the development of chronic sidetracks? Under what conditions can an organization frankly reject those who cannot be maintained in the promotion system? (For instance, does obvious danger in a career activity, such as piloting aircraft, give the authorities the right to be ruthless in getting rid of the unwanted?) On the other hand, under what conditions must the indications of failure be more indirect and subtle? In what ways can the definition of failure be affected and manipulated by the person whose career is directly involved? When, for example, can a person dodge being sidetracked by switching to a different social or organizational career line—different job, different social class aspirations, different institutional treatment program?

BARGAINING OVER THE TIMETABLE

When a career is part of a service or authority relationship, each of the two (or more) groups concerned attempts to structure the same series of events. If the nature of the relationship is more than a unique or fleeting one, each party to the relationship will develop timetable norms that are somewhat different from each other because their goals, their criteria of success or progress, and their conceptions of proper timing are more or less different from each other.

If the relationship is to continue, bargaining and accommodation must take place. The two parties inevitably influence each other's timetables, often simply as a result of anticipating the reactions of the other to given decisions, procedures, rules, or other actions.

Thus, the parent attempts to some extent to impose upon his children his conception of the proper timetable of development, but he must make compromises in response to the spoken and unspoken pressures from his children and his anticipation of how they will feel about the demands that he will make on them. At the same time, children are trying to do some things before they are expected to or allowed to and are trying to avoid doing some other things at the time when they should. The children too modify some of their behavior and some of their pressures so as to avoid conflict with the parents. Thus both parents and children are constantly making compromises about the times when they believe certain events or stages of development should occur.

Of course, there are limiting cases where the room for bargaining over the timetable is narrowed to the vanishing point. Where we have the imposition of a standardized timetable as a massive bureaucratic procedure—as in compulsory military service—this limit is approached. Under what conditions does the highly standardized timetable appear? Certainly, the degree of control plays a part. The controlling authority must have the power to impose a timetable without compromise. Not only must the draftee serve his time whether he likes it or not, but his superiors usually have no power to modify the total time or its sequence except under certain specific circumstances (e.g., certain kinds of illness). Giving the underdogs' superiors discretionary power to modify their subordinates' career timetables immediately opens the door to wholesale bargaining.[7]

---

[7] This point is often recognized by hospital medical directors who try to reduce the pressure for concessions from patients by prohibiting their ward doctors from giving patients passes, privileges, or discharges other than those prescribed by a standardized timetable unless the exception is approved by the director or medical board. The difficulty with this solution for the physicians is that it poses another dilemma for them: it prevents the ward doctor from

However, power to control the underdogs is certainly not the only factor leading to standardized timetables. The degree of uncertainty of outcome plays a part, but it is not clear just what that part is. If the outcome of treatment of disease, training for a job, control of sexual behavior, or the rehabilitation of criminals is highly uncertain, it may seem to be a good reason for considerable leeway in timing the sequence of events in each of these careers and thus promoting a wider area of bargaining between superior and subordinate, professional and client, or two parties engaged in a joint series of acts. However, sometimes the effect is quite the opposite—a standardized timetable is imposed or maintained as a way of avoiding the disruptive consequences of uncertainty and widespread bargaining. Thus, the outcome of academic education in terms of test performance of pupils is highly variable and uncertain, yet the public school system imposes one of the most rigid, unvarying timetables of progress in a career that we can find in our society. Hospital physicians, too, sometimes impose standard time points in areas where uncertainty is greatest: for example, the sequence of giving passes after admission or surgery. Perhaps standardization results from a combination of a high degree of uncertainty and a powerful authority to impose a timetable without compromise. However, this question can only be addressed with more assurance after there have been further studies of career timetables in a variety of areas differing in certainty, power of authority, and perhaps other factors. In any study of a career timetable, there should be an effort not only to determine to what extent and in what ways the timetable is or is not standardized, but also what there is about the career and bargaining situation that produces or prevents standardization.

Another aspect of the timetable that deserves attention is the use of testing points. These, too, must be imposed by an authority

---

exercising his independent expert judgment in treating his patients and thus makes him somewhat less of a physician according to the values held by the medical profession. In fact, this solution can be used only when the ward doctors are internes or residents-in-training or unlicensed foreign physicians working under a restrictive contract.

on subordinates or underdogs and thus become part of the bargaining relationship to the extent that the subordinates can influence the evaluation of their performance or the use to which information about their performance is put. The executive who knows he is being evaluated for a crucial decision about his future promotion potentialities may contrive to control the communication system in such a way that he makes his performance look better than it is to his bosses.

We must be careful, however, to see whether the apparent testing points perform a definite function in affecting the career timetable or whether they are merely empty formalities. A good example of the latter is our public school system, which, despite a standard series of scholastic testing points, promotes and graduates the vast majority of pupils "on time" regardless of performance, on the grounds that it would be psychologically damaging to the pupils to be separated from their age group. Occupations in which seniority reigns supreme may operate in a similar way.

This brings us to another important issue. In the long-term treatment of illness examined in this book, the bargaining process in every case tended to move the length of hospitalization of patients toward the average or norm. Pressure from patients for release increased as they were kept past the expected time, and even physicians came to think of prolonged hospitalization as a reason for considering discharge more favorably. The envy generated when a patient was far ahead of the expected timetable, as well as the physicians' doubts about the credibility of a rapid cure or improvement, had the effect of prolonging the stay of patients whose condition seemed to improve rapidly. The same process seems to be at work in the social and intellectual development of children—rapid developers are often held in check and slow developers are pushed ahead, making them all more "normal." Is this phenomenon common to many other career timetables, and what conditions promote or block such an "averaging" effect?[8]

_____

[8] Remember, too, that the underdogs in a bargaining relationship do not invariably want to speed up the timetable, although the selection of illustrations

Perhaps the most interesting and most important aspect of a study of bargaining over career timetables is the process by which the actual bargaining is conducted. Of course, we have instances where such negotiation is overt and explicit, as in the bargaining between white and Negro groups over a timetable of racial equality. In most cases the bargaining is sub rosa, often explicitly denied, as when a physician says he will not bargain with patients about treatment, a parent says he will not bargain with his children about freedom to go places alone, a prison commissioner says he will not bargain with rioting prisoners about the conditions of parole. In such cases the bargaining goes on without seeming to and sometimes must be hidden to be successful.

Such indirect bargaining becomes a complex process of social interaction. The client, the inmate, the subordinate, the controllee must accumulate information about the careers of others of his kind (and must decide who his kind are) so that he may develop a conception of what his expected timetable is. By observing and comparing notes with his fellows he can build up a dossier of precedents, pressures, and subversive actions that can be used against those who officially control the timetable in an effort to modify the timetable in accordance with his expectations and wishes (which are frequently simply a reflection of the norms of his colleague group). The amount and conditions of access to information about the experiences of his colleagues, the way in which he obtains information, and the use made of this information to modify the timetable are all major foci of the study of bargaining around the career timetable.

At the same time, the professional, the expert, the authority, the controller must decide what an appropriate timetable for his charges is and must defend his decisions against their pressures to change them. He must seem more certain than he really is. He must

---

in this book may have given that impression. Sometimes an effort is made to slow it down either as a whole or, as in the case of the copilots putting off transition school, in selective part in order to increase the chances of success in the long run.

try to hold off special concessions while appearing to give consideration to special circumstances. He too must communicate with his colleagues in order to define "reasonable" points on a timetable, to make an effort to maintain a consistent front against pressure for changes and concessions, and to gain support for decisions that restrict the actions of those over whom he exercises control.

Both controller and controllee, however, must constantly modify their own inclinations in response to the reactions and anticipated reactions of the other party. Strictly unilateral action without regard to the reactions of others may lead to an outcome that is definitely not desired. The patient who pushes too hard to move toward discharge may end by being cut off from treatment; the employee who tries to force promotion may find himself out of a job; the child who tries to extort privileges may be cut off from the affection and protection of his parents. On the other side, the physician who ignores the demands of the patients may completely lose control over them; the employer who will not bargain over promotion may lose his best employees; the parent who tries never to give in to his child may lose the child's affection. Just what are the limits to which one may push one's side of the negotiation without endangering a greater value? This is one of the important decisions that must be made in the bargaining relationship, and the ways in which such decisions are reached can be an important focus for the study of bargaining over the timetable.

INTERACTION OF TIMETABLES

The timetable analyses I have presented in this book were directed toward specific areas or activities that included only part of the lives of many people. That is, they dealt in each case with the one thing that all the people in a group had in common—the treatment of TB or polio or mental disease, work as a pilot or auto assembly plant employee or teacher, getting an education through the school system, fighting for racial equality. The selection of career boundaries is to some extent arbitrary. We select those which suit our purpose. Child development, for example, is a rather broad career category, and for certain purposes we may want to focus on the timetable of subdivisions of child development —linguistic development, sexual development, development of social group formation—recognizing that they are to some degree related and will affect one another. Of course, the selection of career boundaries cannot be completely arbitrary. The category used must have meaning to the people whose behavior is being studied; otherwise, it could scarcely be used as an explanatory device for that behavior.

If one wishes to apply a timetable analysis to the whole of a person's life, he must realize that each person is operating on a number of timetables simultaneously. The amount of pressure the long-term patient brings to bear to influence his treatment timetable may depend on his occupational or family timetables. A man may be a parent concerned with measuring the development of his children in terms of the expectations about child development in his social group and at the same time be a professor measuring his success in his professional career by reference to the expectations of his occupational colleague group. His career stage will affect the school where he chooses to teach, which in turn will affect the kinds of schools, neighborhood, and companions to which his children will be exposed at a given stage of their development. (It may also work the other way around—the stage of development of the professor's children may determine his place of residence, which will partly determine the kind of occupational position he can obtain at a given point in his professional career.) If the focus is on individual development, the interactions between timetables may be of more interest than the separately analyzed career timetables.

A similar approach may be applicable to a process study of families or other small, homogeneous, ongoing social units. Families may have timetables of progress or development, commonly including such major bench marks as the birth, marriage, and death of individual members, social and geographical mobility, the purchase of a home and other major possessions. Developmental cycles of families have frequently been described by anthropologists in studies of primitive groups. The primitive family has usually been regarded as a unitary group, with the developmental timetables of the individual members a well-integrated part of the total family pattern. It is precisely this assumption, however, that will not hold up with regard to our own modern family. (Of course, it often does not hold up in the case of primitive societies either, but the discrepancy is much smaller and often unnoticeable.) For this reason, we must pay more attention to the career timetables of individual family members, the extent to and manner in which they conflict with the total family timetables, and the manner in which the conflicts are resolved. We might also examine the relative influence of the individual timetables on the total family timetable. We may expect, for example, that the husband's occupational timetable will have a major influence, but in many lines of work this may not be true. We may ask whether the housewife-and-mother role can have an important timetable which is not merely a reflection of that of the total family group. Do housewives, as such, have a career? And if so, do they have intercommunicating groups that develop timetable norms for their career role?

Does it make sense to speak of a consumption career, and do interacting groups of consumers develop norms of timetables of consumption? Are there careers of social participation with a timetable of statuses through which the participants expect to move?[9] If so, how do such timetables interact with work and family career timetables? Do some groups of people operate on still other timetables that we have not yet teased out at all? Such issues can be effectively dealt with only when there has been more detailed longitudinal investigation of various spheres of human activity and of the interaction between the spheres.

It may well be possible, and for some purposes useful, to conceive of the life cycle as an interacting bundle of career timetables.

[9] A hypothetical scheme of the interaction of cycles of work, family, consumption, and participation is presented in Harold L. Wilensky, "Life Cycle, Work Situation, and Participation in Formal Associations," in Robert W. Kleemeier, *Aging and Leisure* (New York: Oxford University Press, 1961), especially pp. 227-35.

Recapitulation   2

People try to reduce the uncertainty of what lies ahead of them in time by drawing, when possible, on the experience of others who have gone or are going through the same series of events. As a result of such comparisons, norms develop for entire groups about when certain events may be expected to occur with respect to given reference points. When many people in an interacting group go through the same series of stages or events in a given direction or on the way to a definite and recognizable end-point or series of goals, we speak of this as a "career," of the sequence and timing of events as a "career timetable," and of the consensus of expectations about when the events should occur as the "timetable norms."

Long stretches of time may be made more "psychologically manageable" by being broken up into smaller segments. When the markers used to divide periods of time into segments are also signposts of progress in a given direction, we have the foundation of a career timetable. In retrospect, such signposts become reference points from which further progress may be predicted and measured. The meaning each signpost has for progress through a career develops from communication of experience of those who have passed through the career stages previously. When the conditions of a career undergo a marked change, the reference points may become unclear and less accurately predictive and the search for clues of a timetable structure more desperate. Such clues can never be completely absent because of the consistency and regularity that inhere in the actions and decisions surrounding any career. If new or alternative careers arise beside an older career line, the lack of clarity of the new events and stages may be reduced by making them equivalent to analogous points in the older line.

Each individual uses the timetable norms of the group as a yardstick to measure his own progress. From a comparison of his own rate of progress with the norm he can determine whether he is behind, on, or ahead of schedule. In order to know what norms to apply as a yardstick, the individual must have a model group with which he identifies—a group with whom he believes he closely shares relevant career characteristics and experiences and from whose members he may obtain information about future expectations in his timetable. Individuals sometimes decide at some point that their model group is not the most appropriate one after all or that the conditions of their career have changed sufficiently to make their experiences closer to a different category of career colleagues. In such a case they can switch to a new model group and thus to a new set of timetable norms that will, hopefully, be more accurately predictive.

Even without explicitly switching models, the individual may shift time perspectives during the course of his career. The norms are not usually precise points, but rather ranges of time. At an early stage of his career, a person may focus on the more optimistic end of these ranges and then shift his time perspective ahead as his own career lengthens in time. Also, when a career timetable is rapidly changing as a result of changes in external conditions, we may expect a lag in the norms so that most individuals seem to be chronically ahead or behind schedule.

In every career line, some will fall so far behind that they are no longer in the running. Every career must have some provision for such failures—eliminate them, obscure them, or give them a special status outside the promotion system. The way in which failure is handled will depend on the kind of commitment made to the career incumbents as well as on the conditions under which the failure occurs.

No one is ever completely the helpless pawn of career contingencies. His own actions will have some effect—little in some career lines, great in others—on how nearly he can stay on schedule. Also, he often has some degree of choice in the selection of career lines and of models within any career.

When a career is part of a service, authority, or other noncolleague relationship, each of the two (or more) groups concerned attempts to structure the same series of events. Because the two parties will inevitably differ somewhat in their goals, they will develop timetable norms that differ from each other to some extent. If the relationship is to continue, constant bargaining must go on between the expert, the professional, the authority, the controller on the one hand, and the client, the subordinate, the controllee on the other hand, as each tries to bring the operating career structure closer in line with his own goals. In the course of such bargaining, the two parties influence each other's timetables, often simply as a result of anticipating the reactions of the other to given decisions, procedures, rules, and other actions. One common effect of such a bargaining process is to move individual timetables toward the group norms.

The development of career timetables and timetable norms can be discovered most readily where the career is part of an institutional service structure or part of an occupational job hierarchy. The same concepts might also be applied usefully in areas where the time schedule structure is not so obvious. It might be possible, for example, to examine "consumption careers" or "voluntary participation careers" from this viewpoint. Instead of focusing on the timetables of career lines, one might instead focus on the career experiences of an individual, analyzing his life cycle as the interaction of career timetables. The timetables of progress or development of families or other small, ongoing social units may be amenable to a similar approach. Likewise, larger social units—even whole nations—may be seen as moving through a series of steps toward more distant goals while bargaining with other nations or social units whose interests and timing are in conflict with theirs.

Bibliography

In the body of this book I have given references only for those written works of which I made direct use for illustrative materials, quotations, or ideas. In this bibliography are provided some selected references to works that give background information on, or wider extension of, some of the points touched on in the text. A few of these will also be found in foot-note references where I made specific use of them; the majority are listed in this book only in this bibliography.

PREFACE

Becker, Howard S., 1958. "Problems of Inference and Proof in Participant Observation," *American Sociological Review,* 23 (December), 652-60.
   Discusses the nature and process of making inferences from information accumulated through observational techniques.

Becker, Howard S., and Geer, Blanche, 1957. "Participant Observation and Interviewing: A Comparison," *Human Organization,* 16 (Fall), 28-32.
   Details the advantages of the observational approach in the study of social interaction.

Whyte, William Foote, 1955. *Street Corner Society.* Chicago: University of Chicago Press. Appendix: On the Evolution of "Street Corner Society."
   A highly personal statement of the experience of an investigator who lived in his research setting for an extended period and got his material by hanging out with his "subjects."

CHAPTERS 1 AND 2

MacDonald, Betty, 1948. *The Plague and I.* Philadelphia: J. B. Lippin-cott Co.
   This delightful tale of life in a tuberculosis sanitarium written by a talented ex-patient gives the flavor of hospital existence from the patient's point of view as no social science work has been able to do.

Roth, Julius A., 1963. "Information and the Control of Treatment in Tuberculosis Hospitals," in *The Hospital in Modern Society,* Eliot Freidson (ed.). Glencoe, Ill.: The Free Press.
   Describes the way in which patients obtain information about their

condition, treatment, and hospital life; how the staff obtains information about the patients and their conditions; and how this information is used by each in an effort to gain his own goals.

CHAPTER 3

Balint, Michael, 1957. *The Doctor, His Patient, and the Illness*. London: Pitman Medical Publishing Co. Ltd.

This book presents another area of doctor-patient bargaining. It describes how a general practitioner's diagnosis results from negotiation between patient and doctor in which the patient makes "offers" of various illnesses that the doctor may accept, reject, or modify until the two parties settle down to a definite "organized" illness.

Farber, Maurice L., 1944. "Suffering and Time Perspective of the Prisoner," Part IV of Kurt Lewin *et al., Authority and Frustration*. Iowa City, Iowa: University of Iowa Press.

The prisoner calculates what his sentence should be in terms of "justice." It is analogous in many respects to patients' notions about the proper time for discharge from the hospital.

Freidson, Eliot, 1960. "Client Control and Medical Practice," *American Journal of Sociology*, 65 (January), 374-82.
——, 1962. "Dilemmas in the Doctor-Patient Relationship." In *Human Behavior and Social Processes*, Arnold M. Rose (ed.). Boston: Houghton Mifflin Co.

These two papers discuss the nature and handling of conflict between physicians and patients in voluntary practice.

CHAPTER 4

Becker, Howard S., and Strauss, Anselm L., 1956. "Careers, Personality, and Adult Socialization," *American Journal of Sociology*, 62 (November), 253-63.

Presents a broad framework of the conditions of occupational careers in the context of other aspects of the life cycle, including the pacing and timing of career changes and the definition and effects of failure.

Chinoy, Eli, 1955. *Automobile Workers and the American Dream*. New York: Doubleday and Co.

Discusses the effects of lack of upward occupational mobility on the auto factory worker's job and off-job behavior, aspirations, and plans.

Davis, W. Allison, and Havighurst, Robert J., 1947. *Father of the Man.* Boston: Houghton Mifflin Co.

A detailed description of the difference between developmental time schedules of middle-class and lower-class children.

Gesell, Arnold L., and Ilg, Frances L., 1943. *Infant and Child in the Culture of Today.* New York: Harper & Bros.

———, 1946. *The Child from Five to Ten.* New York: Harper & Bros.

Gesell, Arnold L., Ilg, Frances L., and Ames, Louise Bates, 1956. *Youth from Eleven to Sixteen.* New York: Harper & Bros.

The three preceding volumes are not only the best known and most detailed descriptions of the events and stages of child development in a temporal sequence from birth onward, but have in turn become references for developmental norms and ranges of normality.

Goffman, Erving, 1961. *Asylums: Essays on the Social Situation of Mental Patients and Other Inmates.* Garden City, New York: Doubleday and Co., Inc. (Anchor Books).

The four papers in this volume contain rich detail on many aspects of life in mental hospitals, as well as in "total institutions" in general, including the inmate-staff bargaining process.

Newcomer, Mabel, 1955. *The Big Business Executive.* New York: Columbia University Press. See especially Chapters 7 and 8.

Warner, W. Lloyd, and Abegglen, James C., 1955. *Occupational Mobility in American Business and Industry.* Minneapolis: University of Minnesota Press. See especially Chapters 5 and 6.

Both these books are reports on large scale surveys of the American business elite. They provide detailed statistical data on business executive career patterns.

CHAPTER 5

Goffman, Erving, 1952. "On Cooling the Mark Out: Some Aspects of Adaptation to Failure," *Psychiatry,* 15 (November), 451-63. Reprinted 1962 in *Human Behavior and Social Processes,* Arnold M. Rose (ed.). Boston: Houghton Mifflin Co.

Uses the model of the confidence man and his victim to analyze a mode of handling and adapting to failure.

Hughes, Everett C., 1958. "Cycles, Turning Points, and Careers." In *Men and Their Work*. Glencoe, Ill.: The Free Press.

A broad view of the human life cycle in a world where the temporal reference points are rapidly changing and often providing poorly defined clues about the stage of life one has reached.

Merton, Robert K., 1957. *Social Theory and Social Structure*. Glencoe, Ill.: The Free Press. Chapter 8: "Contributions to the Theory of Reference Group Behavior" (with Alice Rossi). Chapter 9: "Continuities in the Theory of Reference Groups and Social Structure."

A recent comprehensive statement of the theoretical and applied use of reference group theory in sociology.

Shelling, Thomas C., 1960. *The Strategy of Conflict*. Cambridge, Mass.: Harvard University Press. See especially "An Essay on Bargaining," pp. 21-52.

A detailed analysis of the bargaining process, including a discussion of how apparent weakness sometimes proves to be a bargaining strength.

Shibutani, Tamotsu, 1962. "Reference Groups and Social Control." In *Human Behavior and Social Processes*, Arnold M. Rose (ed.). Boston: Houghton Mifflin Co.

The use of the reference group concept in symbolic interactionist theory.

Thompson, Laura, and Joseph, Alice, 1947. *The Hopi Way*. Chicago: University of Chicago Press. See especially Chapters 1 and 2.

Detailed picture of a society whose days and years move in a cyclic round of events rather than in a forward-moving progression.

Index